"*A Nurse Practitioner's Guide to Smart Health Choices* is about responsibility, risks, and rewards in making healthy lifestyle choices. It is consumer friendly, readable, credible, and doable. Every family needs this guide and reference for health promotion and healthy choices in daily living. It is a bible to good health."

—Loretta C. Ford, Co-founder of the Nurse Practitioner, Dean and Professor, Emerita, University of Rochester, School of Nursing.

• • •

"When a clinician tells you to 'watch your diet and exercise,' *A Nurse Practitioner's Guide to Smart Health Choices* tells you what that actually means in a way the average person can actually understand."

—Carolyn Buppert, NP, JD

• • •

"*A Nurse Practitioner's Guide to Smart Health Choices* captures the essence of the care NPs give. Partnering with a patient is what it is all about. This book gives folks a tool that helps them take charge of their lives, and choose the path to wellness, quality of life, and independence. It is a resource that I will recommend to all my patients and the students I teach. It exemplifies partnering for health at its finest."

—Mona Counts, PhD, CRNP, FNAP, FAANO, President, American Academy of Nurse Practitioners

• • •

"*A Nurse Practitioner's Guide to Smart Health Choices* is about what nurse practitioners do best which is to teach people how to stay healthy and prevent disease. And while nurse practitioners are skilled at treating disease, we recognize that staying healthy is far better than fixing problems once they have developed."

Susan Wysocki, RNC, NP, FAANP, President and CEO,
National Association of Nurse Practitioners in Women's Health (NPWH)

• • •

"NPs, stand up and salute. Carla Mills has written a book to make all NPs proud. *A Nurse Practitioner's Guide to Smart Health Choices* is a well written 'how to' manual for those contemplating a lower-risk lifestyle. Carla captures completely the holistic, integrated orientation unique to NP practice. Included in this tremendous work are the major lifestyle and behavioral causes of disease, disability, and premature death—plus action steps that help you stick to lifestyle changes you choose. This book is a gift to those who truly want to transform their health risks. It belongs on the shelf with other classics on patient empowerment."

— Eileen T. O'Grady, PhD, RN, NP,
Policy Liaison, American College of Nurse Practitioners

• • •

A Nurse Practitioner's Guide to Smart Health Choices

Carla Mills, ARNP
Advanced Registered Nurse Practitioner

with Jamie Shane, CYT
Certified Yoga Teacher

Foreword by Robert Boyd Tober, MD, FACEP
Fellow of the American College of Emergency Physicians

First Edition

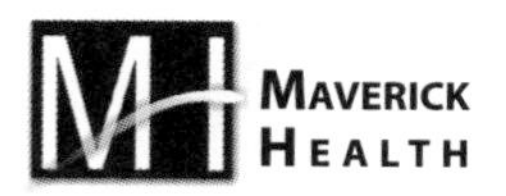

Published by
Maverick Health
12290 Treeline Avenue
Fort Myers, FL 33919
Phone: (800) 595-2315
Email: info@MaverickHealth.com

Printed in the United States of America

Library of Congress Cataloging-in-Publication Data
Mills, Carla.

A nurse practitioner's guide to smart health choices / Carla Mills with Jamie Shane ; foreword by Robert Boyd Tober. -- 1st ed. -- Fort Myers, FL : Maverick Health Press, 2007.

p. ; cm.

ISBN-13: 978-0-9789758-0-7
ISBN-10: 0-9789758-0-4
Includes bibliographical references and index.

1. Health behavior. 2. Well-being. 3. Health education.
I. Shane, Jamie. II. Title.

RA776.9 .M55 2007
613--dc22 0706

Cover Photo by Robert Nelson Photography
Book cover and page design by Jeanie James, Shorebird Media

Disclaimer

This book has been written to provide reliable medical information directly to consumers. It is not intended to replace, but rather add to, care you receive from your primary health practitioner. **Medical practice and medical diagnosis require direct, face-to-face interactions, physical examination, and evaluation of laboratory and diagnostic testing.**

Always seek the advice of a trained health professional before seeking any new treatment regarding your medical diagnosis or condition. Any information received from this book is not intended to diagnose, treat, or cure. It is provided for information purposes only. All data is presented as is, without any warranty of any kind, express or implied. While every effort has been made to provide the highest-quality information possible, we are not liable for its accuracy or for mistakes or omissions of any kind, nor for any loss or damage caused by a user's reliance on information obtained here.

Our goal is to present complex medical information in a simple, understandable, and useful way to non-medical consumers. The information contained here has been derived from an exhaustive review of current medical literature, relying most heavily on evidence-based research and approved national guidelines. It has been compiled and interpreted by a Board Certified Family Nurse Practitioner for the purposes of education only.

The information obtained should not be construed as medical advice but rather as information published for the purpose of enabling consumers to direct self-care activities in a more precise, effective, and goal-directed way.

If you do not wish to be bound by the above, you may return this book to the publisher for a full refund.

For my patients
whose struggles and triumphs taught me what matters.

Note to the Reader

About the Checklists

This book has checklists and fill-in-the-blanks to help you learn about your health. If you do not own the copy you are reading, if you might want to share it with others, or if you checked it out of the library, *please do not mark directly in this book.*

You are granted permission by the author to make copies of the checklists directly out of the book so long as they are for your personal use only.

About the Guidelines/Links

National treatment guidelines are under constant review by professional organizations and are updated periodically. The guidelines and web links in this book are current at the time of publication.

Updates, changes, and additional resources can be found at our website, www.MaverickHealth.com.

Table of Contents

Letter to the Reader

You are invited to come on a journey of self-discovery that will improve your health and leave you with a sense of well-being and confidence. This book will help you uncover your unique health risks and show you how to reduce them. It's important that you know what your health risks are. Health risks are risky because they have no symptoms. You may feel perfectly fine until the day you are diagnosed with a chronic disease or some catastrophic event like a heart attack, stroke, or cancer befalls you. But if you learn what your risks are and use your behaviors to reduce them, you can actually turn these risks into opportunities—second chances—that will both reduce the danger from your risks and improve your health at the same time.

Staying healthy is a *choice* and you make it with your *behaviors*. Understanding medicine helps, too, and you don't have to be a rocket scientist to accomplish that. With the right information and a little motivation, taking charge of your health and healthcare is actually pretty simple. Regardless of your current state of health, better health is waiting for you. Reading this book and working in partnership with your health practitioner will make you an expert on your own health and the kind of healthcare you need.

If you ...

- struggle to control your weight
- smoke
- have high blood pressure
- have high cholesterol
- have diabetes
- have metabolic syndrome (or if you don't know what metabolic syndrome is)
- have heart disease or family members with heart disease
- suffer from stress, anxiety, depression, or fatigue
- want to feel more vibrant, healthy, energetic, and alive

This book is for you.

I've been a Registered Nurse (RN) for more than 20 years and a Nurse Practitioner (NP) for more than 10. From emergency rooms to intensive care units, in home health, rehabilitation facilities, and now in my private practice, I've seen more suffering, grief, disability, and premature death than I can bear to recall. Most heartbreaking of all is that most of these tragic events were preventable; they didn't just come out of nowhere. Uncontrolled health risks were warning signs that had flashed alarms *for years* before the catastrophic events occurred. But my patients didn't see them coming. They didn't recognize their risks or act on them until it was too late. Over and over I have watched the lights of understanding come on, but only *after* something terrible had happened. Knowing that these tragedies could have been prevented is what prompted me to write this book.

I want to lift the mysterious veil of medicine for you. Medicine is not rocket science and it's not magic. Mostly it's common sense. Read this book and you will understand your health and the kind of healthcare you need just as clearly as your health practitioner does. It gives you access to the same treatment guidelines your health practitioner uses. This book is written to be used over and over. Keep going back to it again and again until it is dog-eared and coffee-stained and you know everything in it. It is a friendly guide that will enlighten you about your risks and help you decide what you should do about them. It will inspire you and help you make the behavior changes that will do you the most good based on your own unique risk profile.

Understand at the outset that self-care begins and ends with you ... it doesn't come from your spouse, your health practitioner, or Lady Luck. You give it and you take it. Understanding that, you will finally understand that medicine is powerless to keep you healthy. The best that medicine can do is treat you after you have already become sick. You are the only one who can take care of yourself to keep yourself healthy and well.

I encourage you to take this book home with you. It will change your life.

Carla Mills, ARNP

Foreword

By Robert Boyd Tober, MD

Carla Mills has written a book that could transform the lives of millions of Americans by showing how we can reduce our risks for major disease. During 28 years as an emergency room physician, I have looked in the eyes of more than 100,000 critically ill patients, and, in so many cases, I have seen tragedies that could have been averted by applying the knowledge in this book.

I have told a 39-year-old female who had diabetes that she had to have her leg removed because of the lack of a blood supply and the onset of gangrene. In her own eyes, I saw loss and bewilderment … but only a faint understanding that the cigarettes she so diligently smoked for the past 19 years had destroyed the last remnants of blood flow to her leg.

I have seen confusion in the eyes of a 46-year-old man when I told him he was having a heart attack. Despite his history of high blood pressure, and his own father's early death from cardiac arrest, he thought everything was okay, because up until that last moment, he seemed to feel just fine.

Serious and often fatal health events result when we remain ignorant of our risk factors for catastrophic illness. At times, my patients remind me of high-flying trapeze artists at the circus. Some people choose to put strong nets beneath them. Others are either confident enough, or careless enough to fly through the air (and life) without preparing for a safe landing. Most of the diseases that I treat are the final result of choices in life that sent patients flying through the air with no nets underneath them. Many of those who plummet downward land in the emergency room, which is the final safety net for those lucky enough to reach it.

Carla has written a book that sets the record straight on just how much choice we all have about how healthy we remain throughout our lives. She has carefully detailed for us just how we can all string "nets of safety" beneath us with our lifestyle choices. She shows us where the largest gaps in our own nets are, and where we are at risk for falling through them.

Sadly, our current healthcare system is overwhelmed and fragile. It is a mistake for us to count on this overstretched system to look after us, and it is not likely to get better anytime soon. We must look after ourselves and take matters into our own hands. That is why Carla's book is long overdue and so desperately needed. This wonderful and clinically gifted Nurse Practitioner has created a friendly and comprehensible path for us to follow through a maze of controversies in healthcare.

As a physician facing more than 20 critically ill or dying patients during a busy 10-hour shift each day, my primary task is to figure out exactly what is wrong with a patient on arrival. There is little time or opportunity to communicate to patients how the choices they have made have led to the current crisis. I have to overcome a lifetime of abuses in order to stabilize, and hopefully save, the patient's life. From now on I plan to keep a copy of Carla's book in my black bag. I am going to ask individual patients to read particular paragraphs or chapters while I run to tend to the next patient.

This book should be required reading for every patient and every practicing healthcare provider in America. If everyone carefully followed the lessons taught here, my business in the emergency room would be reduced by 75 percent!

Yes, there will always be accidents. There will always be bad luck. There will always be infectious diseases and unavoidable health problems, but destiny, for the vast majority of us, is a matter of *choice*. Carla's book puts the choice back in your hands.

Robert Boyd Tober, MD, FACEP
Medical Director, Collier County Emergency Medical Services
Medical Director, Neighborhood Health Clinic
Medical Director, NCH Wound Healing Center
Voluntary Professor of Medicine, University of Miami School of Medicine

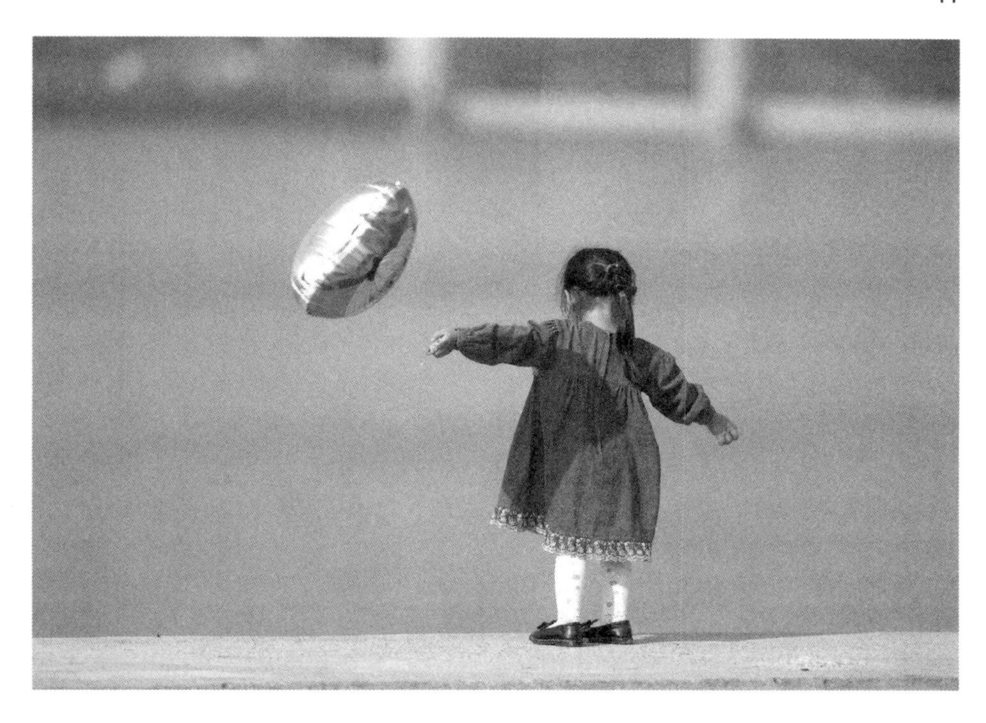

How Is Your Health?

When I was little, my mother used to tie the string of a balloon around my wrist to make sure I didn't lose it. One day, when she deemed me old enough, she put the string into my little hand, and I was entrusted with the care of my own beloved balloon. And guess what happened? Yep, one moment of inattention and it went sailing off into the wild blue yonder, never to be seen again. Tragic.

We can equate my balloon to your health. It could take a lifetime, or just one cosmic moment of distraction and it is gone. Poof. Just like that. But, luckily, unlike my balloon, you can almost always get your health back.

Barring certain conditions, we are all born with a measure of good health, and we live our lives as if this will never change. Your life experience is irrevocably tied to your health. And most of us just don't give this a second thought. But the true nature of health gives you only two choices. Either you control it, steering it with due diligence in the direction you want it to go, or you let it slip away from you.

Most people's understanding of health is fraught with misperceptions, fear, and ignorance. So much of our health today is shrouded in medical mystery. It has been taken from our hands and elevated to a science that the average person cannot understand. Something as simple and basic as health has become mystified to the point where we can barely navigate its course.

This has brought us to a point where we can only define our health in terms of base sensation. Ask people about their health and they will probably answer, "Well, I feel fine." This is the universal human gauge of health. *How do you feel?*

But is feeling fine really an accurate gauge of your health? Can you feel cholesterol gathering in the arteries of your heart? Can you feel high blood pressure? Can you feel rising insulin levels? Can you feel high blood sugar? Can you feel the growth of abnormal cells, say, in your lung from smoking?

No, you cannot. So how can you say with confidence that you are healthy just because you feel okay?

Using this method to determine the state of your health is a dangerous practice, just as ignoring your well-being is the very best way to lose it.

Whether you are in great health or have health problems, this book will show you how to set yourself on a path that will protect not just your present health but your future health, too. It will guide you through common health issues and show you how to take control of them.

This book, *A Nurse Practitioner's Guide to Smart Health Choices,* offers you the opportunity to survey your health status and develop a plan to lower your risks for disease and improve your chances for staying well. Using easy, concrete, and measurable strategies, you can identify and manage many potential health risks. If you will bring your commitment and resourcefulness along, this book will guide you to a place beyond health worries and limitations. It will put you on a path to wellness.

> *But, before you begin, take a moment first and forgive yourself. Discard any regrets and self-blame so that you are free to move forward. Today is yours to create. If you*

are lucky, you will have a tomorrow, too, to create the kind of life and health you want. This book is about learning your health risks and turning them into health chances—chances that give you the best odds for improving your life.

So, what exactly *is* good health and how do you create it?

Good health is so much more than not being sick. Being healthy is about actively and purposefully behaving in ways that leave you stronger, better nourished, less stressed, and more comfortable in your body and mind. Being healthy awards you the physical, mental, emotional, and spiritual capacity for self-actualization and personal dream fulfillment. When you are healthy, you enjoy many benefits. You are hardy and sound in body and mind. You possess vigor, physical and emotional strength, and joyful well-being. Being healthy is a prerequisite to achieving that higher state—wellness.

Using this book, you can devise a plan that will get you back on track. Just knowing you are doing the things you can do will give you peace of mind about your health future. Regardless of your current health status, you really can change the course of your health with your behaviors. *If you will accept this as true,* there is really nothing in your life you cannot transform if you want to enough.

And you do not (and should not) have to give up the things you enjoy to achieve good health. Life without its joys and pleasures is no life at all. You will simply cut back in areas that aren't helping your health and press ahead in areas that will make you healthier. You may be surprised when you discover that your sources of pleasure will adapt to your new desires.

Be proactive. Be involved. Engage in behaviors and activities that reduce the risks that threaten your life. There are no guarantees, of course, but the better you take care of yourself by reducing your health risks, the better your chances are of aging gracefully and well.

It is possible to make staggering changes. The rewards of doing so are huge. But you must first fully understand the answer to one simple question:

How is your health?

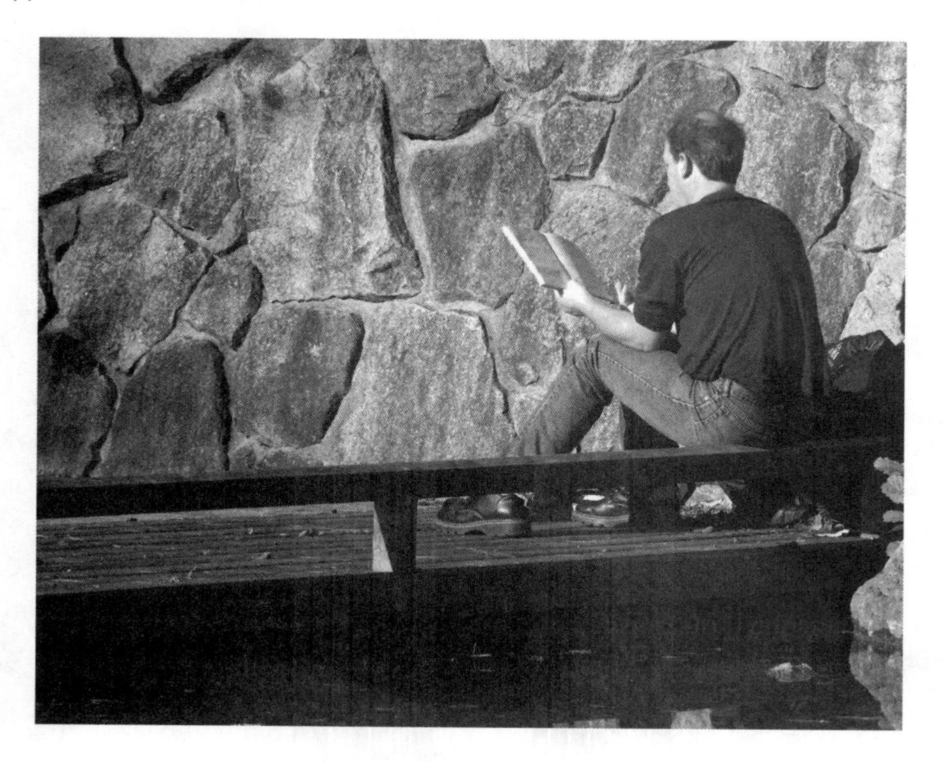

User Guide

In order to make the best use of this book, you will need to know certain things about your health status and have at your fingertips certain measurements. Knowing the following information will give you everything you need to be able to put yourself and your circumstances into the book and take from it what is most meaningful in your particular circumstances.

Most of the following information you can find out for yourself. If you have had recent routine blood tests, you may be able to complete this on your own. If not, your primary health provider or a convenient walk-in clinic can help you. You should also have a complete list of your medications and their doses (including any vitamins or supplements you take) and be familiar with health problems that run in your family.

Body Measurements

Name: ______________________________

Age: ______________________________

Height (inches): ______________________________

Weight (lbs): ______________________________

BMI (see page 210): ______________________________

Waist Measurement (inches): [1] ______________________________

Hip Measurement (inches): ______________________________

Waist/Hip Ratio (Waist inches divided by Hip inches): ______________

Blood Pressure: [2] ______________________________

Heart Rate (# of beats per minute): [2] ______________________________

Blood Tests

A detailed description of each blood test can be found in the Appendix of this book.

Fasting Cholesterol Profile

Total Cholesterol: ______________________________

Triglycerides: ______________________________

HDL: ______________________________

LDL: ______________________________

Complete Metabolic Profile

Sodium: ______________________________

Potassium: ______________________________

Chloride: ______________________________

CO_2: ______________________________

Fasting Glucose (Blood Sugar): ______________________________

---

1 *Tips for measuring waist and hips: measure on bare skin, relax your stomach, don't suck it in, measure your waist at its narrowest point and your hips at the widest point, keep the tape parallel with the ground all the way around, take three measurements at each location and average the three to get the most accurate measurement.*

2 *Tips for measuring blood pressure (BP) and heart rate (pulse): you can check your blood pressure with a home BP monitor, at your local grocery or pharmacy where there are often free BP machines, or by a health professional; your heart rate is measured by counting your pulse (see page 93 for instructions). Both will vary depending on the time of day and your activity level. Take three measurements at different times and on different days to get an average.*

BUN: ____________________

Creatinine: ____________________

Total Protein: ____________________

Albumin: ____________________

Calcium: ____________________

Bilirubin, Total: ____________________

Alk Phos: ____________________

ALT (SGPT): ____________________

AST (SGOT): ____________________

TSH (Thyroid-Stimulating Hormone): ____________________

Complete Blood Count (CBC)

WBC: ____________________

RBC: ____________________

Hemoglobin: ____________________

Hematocrit: ____________________

MCV: ____________________

MCH: ____________________

MCHC: ____________________

RDW: ____________________

Platelets: ____________________

Additional Risk Marker Blood Tests

Homocysteine: ____________________

C-reactive protein (CRP): ____________________

HbA1c (only if you have Diabetes): ____________________

Depression and Anxiety Scales *(If your answers are greater than 3, you may be at risk.)*

Depression: *For the last two weeks, I have felt:*

1-not at all depressed

2-not depressed

3-neither depressed nor not depressed

4-a little depressed

5-more depressed than not depressed

6-very depressed

Anxiety: *In general my stress/anxiety level is:*

1-very low

2-somewhat low

3-normal-neither high nor low

4-somewhat high

5-high

6-very high

Health risks you know you already have:

- ☐ High Blood Pressure
- ☐ High Cholesterol
- ☐ Lack of Exercise
- ☐ Excess Weight
- ☐ Smoking
- ☐ Depression
- ☐ Stress and/or Anxiety
- ☐ Metabolic Syndrome
- ☐ Diabetes
- ☐ Heart Disease
- ☐ Cancer

Okay, now you're ready to find out what it all means.

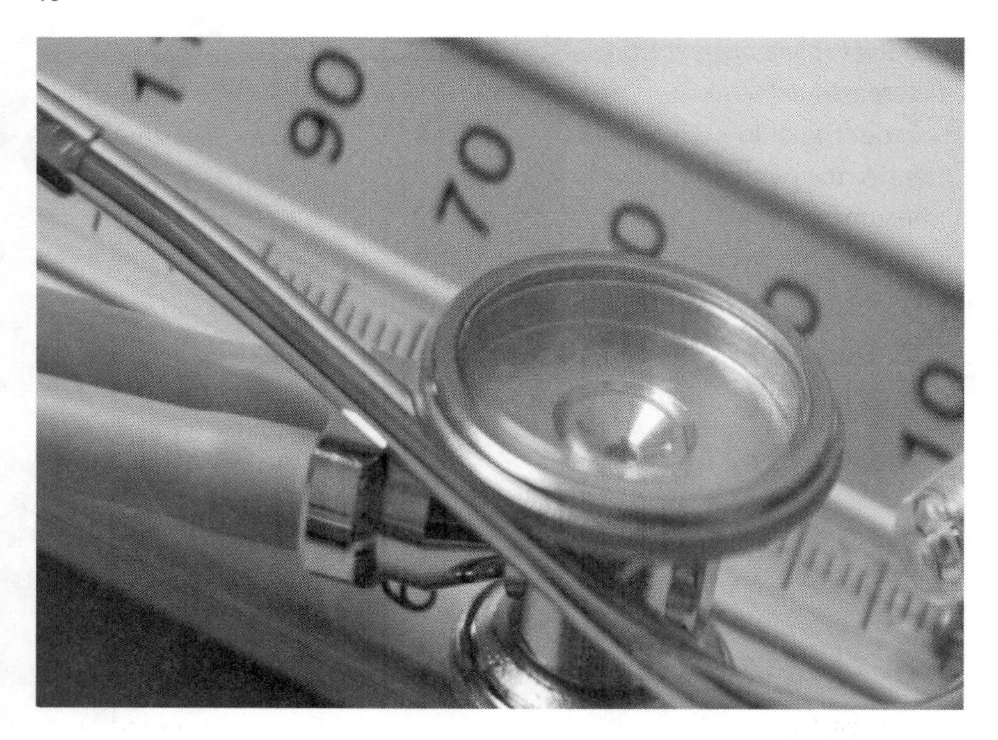

Knowing Is Half the Battle

Nobody wants to discover that the monsters in the closet are real. This is especially true of health monsters. How terrifying to be diagnosed with a serious disease that may require hospitalization, drastic lifestyle changes, and major self-reflection. How much worse to know that had you merely paid attention to the grumblings of the monster before it jumped out of the closet, all that fear might have been avoided.

Once upon a time, disease and premature death were the result of unknown, external causes. They had no reliable treatment or cure. Communicable diseases, unsanitary living conditions, and improper food storage, we know now, were the culprits for much suffering. Diseases like diabetes were death sentences, not preventable and controllable conditions. Thanks to modern science and medicine we have learned how to vanquish most of these former health foes.

However, the tide of disease has changed. Despite our vast knowledge of diagnosis and treatment, we have yet to implement a way to collectively manage the new health monster: *Chronic disease.* Why? Because the diseases that sicken and kill most of us today are caused by our own unhealthy lifestyles. Medicine can't cure us of those; we have to cure ourselves.

Six Leading Causes of Death

According to the Centers for Disease Control (CDC), the following diseases cause seven out of every 10 deaths in the United States. Seventy percent of all deaths in America are caused by one of the following:

- *Heart disease*
- *Cancer*
- *Stroke*
- *Lung disease*
- *Accidents*
- *Diabetes*

Except for accidents, all of these are potentially preventable with healthy lifestyle behaviors.

How you choose to live your life directly affects your health. How you choose to care for your body is directly related to your risk of disease. If you become aware of what you do to yourself, you can greatly reduce your chances of ever developing one of these diseases. Choosing healthy behaviors that reduce risk is the very best way to control the causes of deadly, chronic diseases such as the ones listed above. With the partnership of a health practitioner, these preventable diseases are manageable. But it takes effort. And you must participate actively in your own care.

If you can lay claim to any of the controllable risks below and are doing nothing about it, you are saving up for future illness:

- *High blood pressure*
- *High cholesterol*
- *Excess weight*
- *Lack of exercise*
- *Tobacco and alcohol use*
- *Poor nutrition*

Each of these diseases and the controllable conditions that cause them will be discussed in detail in the chapters that follow. Information on both the best prevention techniques and best medical treatments for each will be included. All the information presented in this book is based on current national treatment guidelines recommended to healthcare professionals by leading health organizations. Depression and anxiety are also included because they, too, can be effectively treated and have a direct impact on your ability to control your other risks.

Do you want good health? Do you aspire to greater wellness? Health will come when you reduce your health risks and take advantage of your health chances. As you go through the process of analyzing your health risks, you will see that everything is connected to everything else. You may find that just one simple behavior change may effectively reduce most of your risks. This book will help you make sure you choose the *right* change for you.

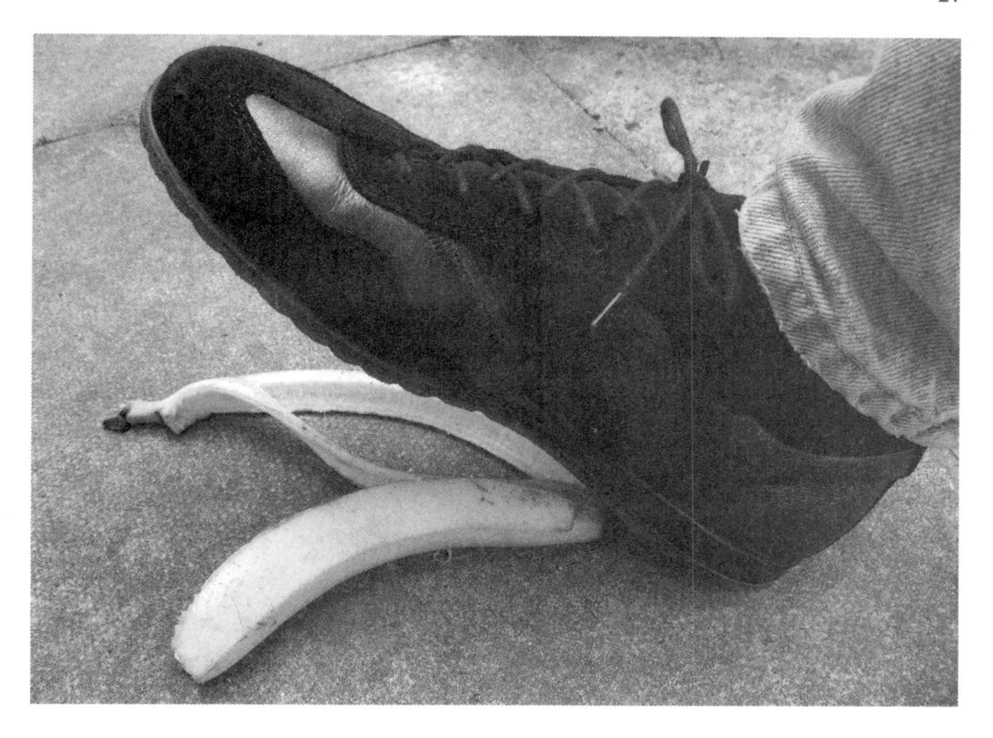

Are You at Risk?

Health risks are universal. Everybody has them. Some you can control and some you can do nothing about. You cannot control your age or your family history. You *can* control your behaviors.

You may have many health risks and never get sick. Or you may have none, and yet still suffer a catastrophic health event like cancer, a heart attack, or stroke. By preparing for things we can control, we are stacking the odds in our favor. Learning about your health risks is the easiest way to acquire essential medical knowledge—*specific* knowledge that is most relevant to your particular circumstances.

Health risks are markers that warn of current or future health problems. They are literally the crystal ball of your health future. They are absolutely the best point at which to intervene to prevent or interrupt the progression of disease. If you focus your medical care on risk factor reduction, it will not only treat current problems, but it will prevent future ones, too. That's how you use your health risks to create second chances.

Are you at risk?

Let's take a moment and answer a few simple questions. They are very broad and general, but they will serve to demonstrate that no matter how well you believe you are taking care of yourself, you still have risk. Just answer yes or no.

Question		
Do you smoke?	❑ Yes	❑ No
Do you drink more than two alcoholic beverages a day?	❑ Yes	❑ No
Do you consume sweets (candy, cookies, cake, pastry) daily?	❑ Yes	❑ No
Does your diet contain processed foods?	❑ Yes	❑ No
Have you been diagnosed with high blood pressure?	❑ Yes	❑ No
Are you more than 20 lbs overweight?	❑ Yes	❑ No
Do you have stress or anxiety?	❑ Yes	❑ No
Do you exercise *less than* 240 minutes a week outside of your work and everyday life?	❑ Yes	❑ No
Have you had long-term sun exposure?	❑ Yes	❑ No
Does anyone in your family have high blood pressure?	❑ Yes	❑ No
High cholesterol? Metabolic syndrome? Diabetes?	❑ Yes	❑ No
Heart disease or cancer?	❑ Yes	❑ No

If you answered yes to even one of these questions, you are in bountiful company.

For quite a while now, western culture has slowly convenienced itself into very unhealthy practices. Mass media marketing of the perfect lifestyle of leisure combined with the abundance of quick and easy food choices have made Americans both overweight and inactive. We are trying to convince ourselves that we don't really have to do anything, and if we wait long enough, whatever we want will be delivered to our door. Is this a lifestyle we want to continue to cultivate? Will it really be able to save us?

No. We are in a state of health emergency. And while there's a lot wrong with health in America, some things have always been right. This is still one of the greatest countries in the world when it comes to the practice of medicine. But our healthcare system is overburdened, insurance companies are growing more difficult to work with, and so patients are being asked to become more self-reliant. Therefore, you have been voted a managing partner in the maintenance of your own personal health. Your health future depends on the actions you take. If you wait until you are sick to think about your health, you will miss chances that might have kept you well if you had acted sooner.

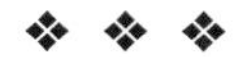

Partnering with Health Professionals

There is simply no better way to determine the state of your health than by visiting a licensed health professional. Not unlike getting your car serviced and its oil changed, or making repairs around the house, a full health screen is part of your responsibility as a body owner. Hoping that your body's health will stand strong for 80-plus years with no tune-ups or checkups along the way is just plain negligence. Keeping your body in tune is considerably easier than fixing it once it is broken—and much cheaper, too. An ounce of prevention really is worth a pound of cure. And it's usually less painful.

Potentially deadly conditions such as colon, prostate, breast, and cervical cancer can all be prevented with regular health screenings. A colonoscopy can find pre-cancerous colon polyps that, when removed during the procedure, cure colon cancer before it even *becomes* cancer. Regular PAP smears for women and digital rectal exams for men can detect cervical and prostate cancers early when they are most treatable. Mammograms can detect breast cancers before they spread.

> *Health screenings give you the opportunity to establish a real baseline understanding of your health position. They inform you of the behaviors you need to cultivate. They also help nurture a trusting relationship with your health practitioner.*

If you only seek healthcare when you are sick, there is never the opportunity to discuss your health risks in detail or plan your health goals for the future. If you arrive sick, you'll get sick care. If you arrive healthy, you'll get healthcare.

This means that you should partner-up with a health professional. A health professional is an extremely well informed health ally. It is in your best interest to engage at least one primary healthcare provider to help you navigate the ins and outs of your health.

Healthcare professionals in today's world fall into two basic categories — primary healthcare providers and specialists. Primary healthcare providers oversee your basic health and healthcare needs. They do your routine examinations, order your lab tests, and take care of your acute illnesses and chronic diseases. They are the ones that refer you to specialists when you need them.

> *Cardiologists, gynecologists, surgeons, gastroenterologists, and oncologists are just a few examples of physician specialists. Other healthcare provider specialists include registered dietitians, diabetic educators, physical therapists, chiropractors, social workers, physical trainers, and yoga instructors—to name just a few.*

As medical care has evolved for both the healthy and the sick, it has become more complex. There are a variety of qualified practitioners available and you will likely see many throughout your life. Your primary healthcare provider might be a nurse practitioner (NP), a physician (MD or DO), or a physician assistant (PA). *See the glossary in the Appendix for more information on these types of providers.*

Perhaps you can see now why it is valuable to have a primary care provider who can act as both quarterback and cheerleader for all your healthcare needs. You should feel comfortable talking over anything with your primary health provider, and he or she should be able to advise and either treat your problem or direct you to a specialist who can.

The best provider-patient relationship is a *partnership* in which both parties bring their own knowledge and experience together to solve problems. This is different from healthcare in the past when a doctor was the boss of everything and made all the decisions. Patients just left doctoring to the doctors. Today, everyone's roles are changing. Modern healthcare offers many choices. Patients now have the option and the added responsibility to investigate all of their healthcare possibilities. Deciding what provider will give you the best care depends on the health problems you have and what you want to do about them. It is your duty to be informed, to understand your care provider's opinion, and *then to make decisions that are right for you. You simply must participate* even if that means enlisting the help of a family member or advocate. There is too much at stake if you do not.

> *Openness and honesty about your beliefs and behaviors is critical to your success in working with any healthcare professional. If you don't want, don't believe in, or can't afford a recommended treatment or medication—say so. You should always feel you can be completely honest. You will be rewarded for your truthfulness by being offered ideas and strategies that are consistent with what you want.*

The chosen treatments will have a better chance of working if they are agreeable and understandable to you. The heart of any partnership is an understanding of what each partner brings to the relationship. Your health practitioner is in charge of the *medical and medication management* of your health problems. You are in charge of the *behavioral aspect* of health risk reduction.

The road to good health is easier together

Together, the two of you can embark upon a plan to first discover and then manage your health risks. We can no longer afford to remain blissfully ignorant of the connection our behaviors have to our health. We cannot believe that sticking our collective heads in the sand convinces risk to fly right by. As comforting as it would be to plop responsibility for our health into someone else's hands, that is simply not a feasible option.

> *It is time to take responsibility. You create your risks. But once you know what they are, you can turn each one into*

a chance. Where risk threatens harm, chance offers new opportunities.

Not all risks are equal, and some symptoms may never present themselves. But that doesn't mean that the risks don't exist. Most of the health risks we will talk about do their damage over years and years, and they do so *without causing any symptoms.*

As you go through this book, learn which risks you should be concerned about *in your particular case.* Learn how to manage your risks and how to reduce them. You will find out that inherent in every risk is a chance—something you can *do* that will not only lower your risk, but will improve your life in positive, health-enhancing ways.

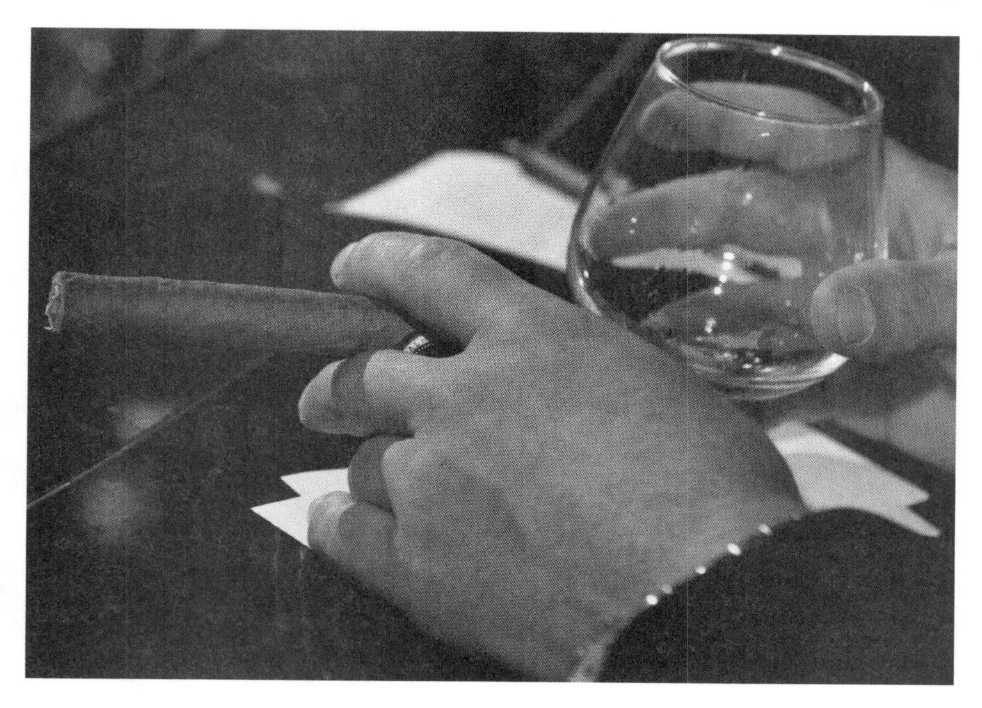

What Are Your Risks?

Heart Attack and Stroke

These are the two leading causes of death and they are a direct result of how we live our lives. If they aren't a concern to you, they probably should be. Of all the causes of death in America, heart disease is number one and stroke is number three (all types of cancer combined are number two). Stroke causes the most long-term disability, too.

Everything in this book, everything your health practitioner does, all the national guidelines and recommendations as well as the hopes of your spouse, family, and friends are intended to make sure that you never suffer either one of these. Your family's and your own health history play an important role, but you are the one with the power of prevention.

If you already have been diagnosed with some form of cardiovascular disease (CVD), you are not alone. About 60 million Americans have one or more forms of cardiovascular disease. CVD claims almost as many lives each year as the next seven leading causes of death combined. It accounts for one-third of all deaths in the United States every year. We all need to respect our risk here and think a little more about our futures and less about our short-term gratifications—before it's too late.

Are you at risk?

Answer yes or no to the things that put you at greatest risk for suffering a heart attack or stroke.

Do you smoke?	❑ Yes	❑ No
Do you have high blood pressure?	❑ Yes	❑ No
Do you have high cholesterol?	❑ Yes	❑ No
Are you overweight?	❑ Yes	❑ No
Do you not exercise?	❑ Yes	❑ No
Do you have metabolic syndrome?	❑ Yes	❑ No
Do you have diabetes?	❑ Yes	❑ No
Do you have a lot of stress and anxiety in your life?	❑ Yes	❑ No
Do heart attacks and strokes run in your family?	❑ Yes	❑ No

Notice that, except for your family history, every other risk is under your control. Are you doing all you can?

If you do suffer a heart attack or stroke, it is by no means a death sentence. Modern medicine has more to offer for these acute life threatening conditions than in almost any other area of medicine. There really are miracle cures available. The trick is you have to recognize what is happening, know what to do, and get to the proper care in time. Treatments for heart attack or stroke must be started *in a hospital* and must begin *within minutes of the detection of symptoms.* Any delay could cost you your life or result in a permanent disability. Recognizing what is happening and acting quickly is essential.

Heart Attack or Myocardial Infarction

In a heart attack, there is a blockage of one or more of the coronary arteries that surround the heart muscle and keep it supplied with blood. If the blood flow is not restored quickly there will be permanent damage to the heart muscle.

If the area of the heart that doesn't get blood is small and the blockage doesn't last long, you will survive. But the part of your functioning heart muscle that didn't get blood will be replaced by scar tissue. Scar tissue will not stretch and pump blood as effectively as healthy heart muscle will. The extent and location of the blockage will determine what your heart function will be like after the attack is over. If the area of the heart that is blocked is large enough and the blockage lasts too long, your heart muscle will not be able to pump blood and you will die from heart failure.

Heart Attack Symptoms

- **Chest pain** (it may be gripping, or feel like pressure, or a dull ache). It may radiate or travel to the neck, shoulders, or left or both arms. People sometimes describe chest pain from a heart attack as feeling like an "elephant sitting on my chest." Some people don't recognize chest pressure as pain and so ignore it. That is very dangerous.
- **Shortness of breath or difficulty taking a deep breath.**
- **Abdominal pain that is often described as "heartburn."**
- **Nausea,** sometimes with vomiting, sometimes not.
- **Sweating that is not associated with heat or exertion.** Feeling cold and clammy while at rest or with only minimal exertion is a symptom of heart attack, particularly if accompanied by any chest discomfort.
- **Dizziness.**
- **Blackouts or fainting.**
- **Fatigue.**
- **Pounding heart or feeling of change in heart rhythm.**
- **Feelings of panic or anxiety.**

Sometimes there is nothing more than a feeling of indigestion or "heartburn" with no other symptoms. Sometimes there are no symptoms at all. This is called a "silent" heart attack.

Symptoms of heart attack are often *denied* or ignored. This is very dangerous and results in many unnecessary deaths.

Women's Symptoms of Heart Attack

Women do not get the same symptoms that men do during a heart attack. The classic chest pain or pressure is often absent in women. Whereas men describe the chest pain of a heart attack as feeling like "an elephant sitting on my chest," women may only experience a "mouse" sitting on theirs. As a result, women often do not seek care quickly enough to receive the best treatments (which, remember, are time-driven).

- **General malaise.**
- **Stomach upset or indigestion** that is not relieved with vomiting.
- **Back or abdominal pain.**
- **Flu-like symptoms.**
- **Shortness of breath.**
- **Dizziness.**
- **Fatigue.**
- **An odd or "not right" feeling.**

Women may even have no symptoms at all. This is called a "silent" heart attack.

Stroke or Brain Attack

A stroke is called a brain attack because the same type of event occurs as in a heart attack, only it occurs in the brain. Certain parts of the brain control specific functions of the body. Speech, balance, and muscle control of various parts of the body are each controlled at specific locations in the brain.

As in a heart attack, the parts of the brain that don't get blood because of a stroke become damaged. The handicaps that result from a stroke depend on what part of the brain is affected. For example, a stroke in the speech center of the brain will create speech handicaps; a stroke in the part that controls the left side of the body will cause left-sided paralysis, and so on.

A transient ischemic attack (TIA) is a "mini-stroke." Its symptoms last a short time and resolve completely on their own without treatment. If you experience a TIA, it is a serious warning, and you should be evaluated in an emergency room or follow up promptly with your health practitioner. Sometimes it's a warning of an impending stroke. With prompt treatment, some people recover completely from a stroke. Others are left with permanent disabilities.

Symptoms of a Stroke or Brain Attack

- **Sudden onset of weakness or numbness** of the face, arm, or leg (usually on one side of the body).
- **Sudden dimness of vision, double vision, or vision loss** (especially in one eye).
- **Sudden confusion.**
- **Sudden difficulty speaking or understanding speech.**
- **Sudden severe headache without obvious cause.**
- **Sudden unexplained dizziness, unsteadiness, balance problems, or falls.**
- **Collapse or loss of consciousness.**

What to Do if a Heart Attack or Stroke Occurs

Do NOT Delay—Call 911

The best way to find out if your symptoms are a heart attack or stroke is to go to your nearest emergency room.

When these attacks occur, minutes count! Your best chance for survival and prevention of damage to your heart or brain is to get to the emergency room within 60 minutes of the onset of your symptoms—sooner if you can. *Every minute counts.* Some treatments cannot be used if you arrive more than 90 minutes after your symptoms started.

- **Call 911** and tell them you think you are having a heart attack or stroke.
- Go to the nearest emergency room by ambulance immediately. Do **not** drive yourself or have a family member drive unless an ambulance cannot get to you.

- Do **not** wait to call your medical practitioner.
- Do **not** take time to consult friends or family.
- Do **not** "wait and see" if your symptoms will go away.
- Do **not** let fear or denial delay you. It could cost you your life.

If you have symptoms of an acute heart attack—chest pain, nausea, vomiting, sweats, anxiety, dizziness, or indigestion—325 mg of aspirin at the time of the symptom's onset may be life-saving (if you have chewable baby aspirin in the house, chewing four of them is better than swallowing them because they get in your bloodstream faster—so is chewing plain aspirin instead of swallowing). Call 911 first *and then chew 325 mg of aspirin.*

There is life after heart attack or stroke. But it will require care and diligent attention. You will be advised to follow all the advice that is outlined in this book. So how about starting right now to reduce your risk?

Cardiovascular Disease

Heart attacks and strokes are caused by cardiovascular disease (CVD). CVD is the number one killer of Americans. This has been so for more than 100 years. Someone in America dies from some form of cardiovascular disease every 33 seconds. That is truly terrifying.

But guess what? Because this disease is most often the result of behavior, if you will have the courage to stare down your risks and learn how CVD works, you can chase it off.

CVD is disease in the heart and blood vessels. Blood is pumped by the heart and travels through the body in arteries and veins. It travels in a constant, necessary flow. No part of our body can live without blood because it carries the oxygen and nutrients needed for life. Interrupted blood flow that is not quickly restored causes tissue death.

CVD can occur anywhere in the body that blood flows. ***How*** it affects the body depends on ***where*** it occurs. All forms of CVD develop from the same process: atherosclerosis or arteriosclerosis (commonly called "hardening of the arteries"). It is caused by one or more risky conditions whose effect on the body results in blood flow interruptions to vital organs. The more cardiovascular risk factors a person has, the greater the risk of suffering a cardiovascular accident.

Cardiovascular risk is highest in individuals who already know they have cardiovascular diseases such as coronary artery disease, carotid artery disease, renal artery disease, peripheral vascular disease, or aortic aneurysm. Risk in people with diabetes, metabolic syndrome, and insulin resistant syndrome (pre-diabetes) is equal to the risk in those who already have CVD. That is why diabetes and metabolic syndrome are considered "cardiovascular risk equivalents."

Are you at risk?

Have you ever had a heart attack or stroke?	❑ Yes	❑ No
Have you ever been diagnosed with narrowing of the arteries in the neck or legs?	❑ Yes	❑ No
Are you a male over 45?	❑ Yes	❑ No
Are you a female over 55 or postmenopausal?	❑ Yes	❑ No
Do you have diabetes?	❑ Yes	❑ No
Do you have metabolic syndrome?	❑ Yes	❑ No
Do you have high blood pressure?	❑ Yes	❑ No
Do you have high cholesterol?	❑ Yes	❑ No
Do you smoke?	❑ Yes	❑ No
Do you exercise less than 240 minutes a week at your target heart rate?	❑ Yes	❑ No
Is your Body Mass Index greater than 25?	❑ Yes	❑ No
Do you have any family history of cardiovascular disease, high blood pressure, high cholesterol?	❑ Yes	❑ No
Has anyone in your family had a heart attack at age 55 or younger?	❑ Yes	❑ No
Do you have a lot of stress and anxiety in your life?	❑ Yes	❑ No
Do you consume more than two alcoholic beverages per day?	❑ Yes	❑ No
Do you now, or have you ever used cocaine?	❑ Yes	❑ No
Do you have sickle cell anemia?	❑ Yes	❑ No

If you answered yes to any of the questions above, read on. You are at risk.

Types of Cardiovascular Disease

- **Coronary Artery Disease** (also called CAD) is caused by either a spasm (constriction) or a blockage of one or more coronary arteries, which are the vessels that wrap around and feed the heart muscle. A blockage may occur gradually over years because of a buildup of fat and cholesterol. Or it can occur suddenly when a piece of plaque breaks off from a vessel wall and lodges in the artery, stopping blood flow through it. This interruption in blood flow to the heart muscle is what causes a heart attack.
- **Carotid Artery Disease** is a blockage of one or both of the large carotid arteries that are on both sides of the neck. These large vessels provide blood to the brain. You can feel them when you check your pulse on either side of your Adam's apple. (Don't feel your pulse on both sides of your neck at the same time, though—that can trigger irregular heartbeats.) If the carotid arteries become blocked with fatty cholesterol and plaque, there is risk of plaque rupture and stroke. Over years, these large arteries can gradually become so blocked that surgery is required to clean them out to maintain blood flow to the brain and prevent a stroke. That surgery is called an endarterectomy.
- **Renal Artery Disease** is a narrowing or blockage of the large arteries that pump blood through the kidneys. The kidneys receive the largest blood flow of any part of the body. About one liter of blood per minute is pumped through the kidneys. The kidneys' job is to filter all the blood in the body and maintain the body's proper internal environment. Kidney function is very complicated. The kidneys do much more than just make urine. They are vital organs. You can live without one kidney, but you can't live without both. Kidney (or renal) failure causes death. Because of the large volume of blood pumped and the size of the arteries, blockage of the renal arteries by atherosclerosis can cause high blood pressure, thus increasing the risk of stroke.
- **Peripheral Vascular Disease** (also called PVD) is blockage in the blood vessels of the legs and arms. A condition called *claudication*

occurs when leg pain develops with walking. That happens because not enough blood is flowing to the legs. Walking, like all exercise, increases the body's need for blood and oxygen in body tissues. Without enough blood (and therefore oxygen) flowing to the muscles of the legs, pain develops. People with claudication have to stop and rest until the pain goes away. When the leg muscles rest they need less blood and oxygen, so the pain goes away and walking can resume. The name for this is *intermittent claudication*. It is another type of cardiovascular disease.

- **Aortic Aneurysm** is a bulging of the wall of the aorta, the largest blood vessel in the body. The aorta runs from behind the heart in the chest down into the abdomen and branches off to smaller vessels that run down the legs. The bulging of the wall of the aorta causes it to become thin and at risk of rupture, much like a balloon that is filled with too much air. It is not known what causes an aortic aneurysm, but risk factors for it are high blood pressure, smoking, and high cholesterol. An aortic aneurysm that ruptures is a life-threatening medical emergency that can cause sudden death.

Screening for Risks

Helping you determine to what extent you are at risk for CVD involves getting some routine screening tests done and reviewing your risks with a health professional.

> *If you are 45 and male, 55 and female, a smoker, a diabetic, have ever had chest pain, or are thinking of beginning a vigorous exercise program, you should to talk to your health practitioner about your CVD risks.*

Whether you feel any symptoms or not, it is in your best interest to have some blood work done and get a physical exam. Your practitioner may advise additional screening tests to detect hidden CVD depending on your current condition and your medical history.

CVD is caused by the way we live and by our genes. We can't do anything about our genes, but we have total control over the way we live. This book is all about using healthy behaviors (and medications, too, if they are needed) as weapons that will reduce your health risks and extend your life and your health.

Prevention by risk reduction along with tight control of any forms of cardiovascular disease you already have is your best insurance against sudden death or disability from a catastrophic health event.

Take every tip that's offered throughout this book and make it your own. Following that course will help you overcome your fears, give you fortitude, and give you the healthiest life you can have.

Diabetes

Diabetes is considered a "risk equivalent" to cardiovascular disease (CVD) because of the damage it causes to the blood vessels in the body. It is increasing at such alarming rates that the Centers for Disease Control (CDC) is calling diabetes an epidemic in the United States.

Twenty-one million Americans are living with diabetes, and it is estimated that six million people have the disease but don't even know they have it. One million new people are diagnosed with diabetes every year. Another 41 million others have metabolic syndrome or pre-diabetes (that's our next topic).

Diabetes is the sixth leading cause of death in America. It is predicted that the number of people with diabetes will grow to more than 30 million in the next 25 years. It used to be a disease that developed later in life, but at the time of this writing, the largest increase in the disease today is among those aged 30 to 39.

The CDC reports that from 1990 to 1998 diabetes increased 70 percent in this age group alone! Because of the high incidence of complications associated with diabetes, the younger you are when it is diagnosed, the higher your risk of developing serious health problems sooner or later. The alarming increase in diabetes is directly linked to lack of exercise, excess weight, and poor

> *diet. Though it is partly genetic, it is most often brought on by poor lifestyle behaviors.*

Diabetes is caused by *too much sugar* (glucose) in the blood. The sugar is trapped in the bloodstream (blood vessels) and can't get into the body's cells where it is needed for energy.

Food is fuel for the body, just like gas is fuel for a car. If you run out of fuel, you can't go any farther until you refill the tank. The type of fuel our bodies use is sugar (glucose). Glucose is the simplest form of sugar and is obtained from digesting (breaking down) food. All types of foods (not just sweet foods) are broken down to glucose. It is the form of energy our bodies use. In order to use glucose for energy, the body must somehow move it out of the bloodstream and get it into the cells.

Glucose gives cells the energy to do their work. Hair cells grow hair, heart cells pump blood, lung cells take oxygen from the air that is breathed, stomach cells digest food, and so on.

Insulin is the chemical transporter that carries glucose out of the blood and into the cells where it can be used to do work. It is a hormone made by our bodies in the pancreas, a fish-shaped organ in the abdomen. In diabetes the problem is either *insufficient* insulin from the pancreas or insulin *insensitivity*. If the cells become insensitive to insulin (usually because of being overweight) the glucose can't get inside the cells to do its work. It is left floating around in the blood. High sugar in the blood is a dangerous condition because it damages blood vessels.

Are you at risk?

Are you overweight?	❑ Yes	❑ No
Do you not exercise?	❑ Yes	❑ No
Is your fasting blood sugar higher than 100 mg / dl?	❑ Yes	❑ No
Is your hemoglobin A1c higher than 6?	❑ Yes	❑ No
Have you had a glucose tolerance test that measured greater than 130 mg / dl?	❑ Yes	❑ No
Do you have a family history of diabetes?	❑ Yes	❑ No
Are you on diabetes medication?	❑ Yes	❑ No
Do you have type 1 diabetes, diagnosed before age 30?	❑ Yes	❑ No

Have you been diagnosed with type 2 diabetes?	❑ Yes	❑ No
Did you have gestational diabetes with pregnancy?	❑ Yes	❑ No
Did you give birth to an infant weighing greater than 9 pounds?	❑ Yes	❑ No
Are you Native American, Asian American, African American, Hispanic, Pacific Islander, or any combination thereof?	❑ Yes	❑ No

If you answered yes to any of these questions, read on. You are at risk.

The most common form of diabetes is diabetes mellitus type 2, or non-insulin-dependent diabetes. It is also called adult-onset diabetes. There are two types of diabetes, but it is type 2 diabetes that has become epidemic in our country. Today even our children are getting adult-onset, type 2 diabetes.

In type 2 diabetes, the pancreas is making insulin, but the cells have become insensitive to it—usually because a person is overweight. The pancreas keeps making more and more insulin to try to control the high sugar in the blood, but eventually the insulin-making cells burn out. That is when type 2 diabetes develops.

Type 2 diabetes can be *prevented* if it is detected and treated early. Don't wait until your blood sugars are already too high before you deal with the possibility of diabetes, or you'll lose your chance to prevent the disease.

Excess weight, poor diet, and lack of exercise are all risks that you create with your lifestyle that can provoke this difficult disease. Sometimes it can be reversed with weight loss, proper diet, and exercise. Studies have proven lifestyle changes are really effective at controlling diabetes. But once full-blown diabetes has developed, pills and even insulin are usually required.

The other type of diabetes is called *diabetes mellitus, type 1* or *insulin-dependent diabetes*. This is an uncommon form of diabetes, accounting for only 5 percent to 10 percent of all cases. The only way to treat it is with insulin injections and these are required for life. This type of diabetes usually begins in childhood or adolescence (it used to be called juvenile-onset diabetes). Type 1 diabetes is believed to be caused by a trigger that affects genetically susceptible individuals. That trigger might be a virus, a toxin, or something in the environment. What is triggered is the destruction of the cells in the pancreas that make insulin. After 80 percent to 90 percent of these beta cells have been destroyed, diabetes type 1 and its associated high blood sugar develop in the body.

So why is diabetes so dangerous?

Over time, diabetes causes damage to the body's vital organs. As glucose circulates around in the bloodstream, it causes damage when it gets into tight spaces. That's because, in comparison to other particles in the body, glucose is very big in size. Imagine a big bowling ball rolling through a lady's hairnet. When it reaches areas where the vessels are tiny and fine (like the hair net), it blows them out. It's not hard to imagine the damage that can be done as that big particle blasts through the small blood vessels.

The areas of the body that have the finest, smallest vessels are where damage from diabetes is most common.

These areas are:

- Arteries of the heart (diabetes can lead to heart attack).
- Vessels in the brain (diabetes can lead to stroke).
- Kidneys (diabetes can lead to kidney failure).
- Retina of the eye (diabetes can lead to blindness).
- Small vessels in the skin, particularly hands and feet (diabetes can lead to poor circulation, erectile dysfunction, skin ulcers that do not heal, and amputations) .
- Nerve cells, which can lead to chronic pain or loss of sensation in the legs (called peripheral neuropathy) .
- Impaired digestive movement in the stomach and intestines (called gastroparesis).
- Fetal development (diabetes can lead to birth defects or overly large infants).

Furthermore, diabetes can create a host of other, smaller health risks. High blood sugar can lead to:

- Carpal tunnel syndrome
- Fungal and bacterial infections
- Tooth and gum disease
- Poor wound healing

Because glucose is food for energy, not only does it fuel people, but it provides food for germs, too. When someone with high blood sugar gets a wound or sore (often on the feet) and germs get there—what a feast! The person's blood flowing to the area is so sweet and full of sugar that the germs stay there and have a great picnic; killing them off can be very hard. Thus, high blood sugar results in the increased risk of infection in diabetics.

Diabetes is dangerous for all the reasons listed above. It is scary because it has no symptoms until it is dangerously out of control. Most people who develop type 2 diabetes have blood sugars that are elevated but not so high that they have symptoms or even know they have the condition unless they get routine blood tests. By the time symptoms do occur blood sugars are *way* out of control. Many people go for years with high blood sugar and never know it.

If there is too much sugar in your blood and it is unable to get into your cells, you are actually starving. The food for energy simply can't get where it needs to go. Because of this, three very bad things begin to happen.

- **Hunger and Weight Loss.** While you may think it is good you are losing weight, you are actually accumulating poisons in your body called ketones. You lose weight even when you eat more. That's because you can't use the sugar trapped in your blood, so you start breaking down muscle and fat for energy. If your diabetes remains untreated, you can develop a life-threatening emergency called diabetic ketoacidosis. This serious form of uncontrolled diabetes poisons you, and is detectable by a fruity odor to your breath. That is followed shortly by mental confusion, coma, and death.
- **Increased Urination.** You are urinating large amounts because it's the only way your body can get the sugar out of your blood. If your urine is tested it will be filled with sugar. By the time you have sugar in your urine, your blood sugars are *way* too high.
- **Increased Thirst.** Because you are urinating large amounts you are dehydrated. That triggers your thirst response and makes you thirsty even though you are drinking large quantities of fluids.

If you have any of the above symptoms, get to your healthcare provider as soon as possible.

You should have a blood sugar test done. Even if you have none of the symptoms, you should still have a blood sugar test. This simple life-saving test can get you on the prevention path before you need to get in the treatment lane.

And even if you need medications or insulin to control your blood sugars, you should not dismiss the value of a lifestyle change to the course of this disease. Whether you are on oral medication, insulin, or a combination of both, you will discover that your successful control of diabetes depends on *what you eat.* The proper foods, in the proper amounts, at the proper times will do more to control your blood sugars than anything else you do.

Many new diabetics hope that their medications will control their blood sugars so they won't have to pay attention to their diet. Unfortunately, it doesn't work this way. *As long as your diet is out of control, your blood sugars will be, too.*

Combining diet and medications to achieve blood sugar control requires knowledge and desire, but control can be achieved. Once your blood sugars become controlled, you will feel better, and you may find that the lifestyle required isn't as hard as you initially thought it would be.

Taking the time and investing the effort to become an expert about your diabetes and your diet is definitely worth it. It is said there is no diabetic diet, just a healthy diet, but you do need to understand how food and blood sugar relate to one another. Detailed teaching about the requirements of a balanced diet for balanced blood sugars is beyond the scope of this book. You are strongly encouraged, at the start, however, to seek education from a registered dietitian, a diabetic educator, the library, or the Internet. You will find a wealth of resources out there if you look for them.

In the meantime, here are some basic meal-planning tips from the American Diabetes Association to help get you started:

- **Eat from all food groups** at each meal and snack. Include carbohydrates, protein, and fat. Protein and fat consumed along with the carbohydrate slows the rise in blood sugar and evens out blood sugar fluctuations.
- **Eat three meals a day** instead of skipping meals or eating one or two larger meals.

- **Try to space meals** about four hours apart to allow your blood sugar to recover before your next meal.
- **Eat a consistent amount of carbohydrates at each meal.** If you are overweight and have type 2 diabetes, 45 grams of carbohydrates at each meal will help you lose weight and control your blood sugar.
- **If you are overweight and have type 2 diabetes, you probably don't need snacks.** Three well-spaced healthy meals a day should control your blood sugar and provide adequate energy.
- Furthermore, you must **lose weight, exercise regularly, control blood pressure and cholesterol, and if you smoke—quit.** This is all critical and must be done. Yet these lifestyle changes and oral medications may not be enough to manage your diabetes. In that case, insulin injections may be required.

About insulin

Different types of insulin vary by how quickly they start working, how long until they reach peak effects, and how many hours they keep lowering your blood sugar.

- **Rapid and short-acting insulins** start lowering blood sugar within 15 to 30 minutes. They are often used in insulin "sliding scales" to quickly reduce blood sugars that are higher than they should be.
- **Medium-acting insulins** are usually taken twice a day and last around 12 hours.
- **Long-acting insulins** last 18 to 24 hours. At the time of this writing, the newest form of long-acting insulin is called *Lantus*. It mimics natural insulin and so has no peak. It is used alone or along with short-acting insulin taken at meals to control blood sugars evenly and avoid wide swings in blood sugar from high to low.

Insulin requires finger-stick blood-testing and regular injections. At the time of this writing, a new insulin that can be inhaled is coming on the market. There are also insulin pumps available that try to mimic the insulin release that would occur in a non-diabetic. Many experienced diabetics who have their diets well controlled prefer these. Your healthcare provider will give you detailed instructions on how to manage this aspect of your care or will refer you to a specialist for advice.

The risk with insulin (and with oral medications, too) is that the blood sugar can go too low (a condition called *hypoglycemia* or *insulin reaction*). The medications prescribed are to take the sugar out of the blood and move it into the cells where it can do work. Because medications remove sugar from the blood, hypoglycemia can occur if meals are skipped or there is stress that increases sugar requirements (like exercise or illness, for example).

Symptoms you may feel with low blood sugar include getting shaky, sweaty, confused, irritable, cold, or hungry. You should check your blood sugar immediately if any of these symptoms occur and consume sugar if your blood sugar is less than 70 mg / dl. The treatment is eating or drinking sugar (like orange juice, milk, sugar, honey, or soda) in order to bring your blood sugar up quickly. Don't go overboard, though. If you overcompensate, your sugars will shoot up too high.

If too much insulin is taken and / or not enough food is eaten, your blood sugar may drop so low that you become confused or even unconscious. This is very dangerous. If you are driving or alone and there is no one there to get sugar into you, you can die from insulin-induced hypoglycemia.

This is a life-threatening emergency. If you can't take sugar by mouth because you are unconscious, paramedics can save your life by giving you sugar through an intravenous line. If you are diabetic and on medications, you should wear a medic alert bracelet, carry a card in your wallet, and tell friends and family members what to do if you become unconscious from low blood sugar.

Diabetes is no joke. It is a very real health crisis, but one that can be managed. It can even be prevented.

Take the time to really examine your health behaviors and weigh them against everything you have learned thus far. Is your apathy really worth the trials you may face as a result? Taking your risks in hand pulls the teeth from your personal health monster and turns it into a house pet.

It is in your power to make changes.

Metabolic Syndrome

Metabolic syndrome is a specific combination of conditions that together create a very high health risk for diabetes, heart disease, vascular disease, sudden heart attack, and stroke. The scary thing about metabolic syndrome (which has also been called *pre-diabetes* and *Syndrome X*) is that many of the people who have it have never even heard of it.

Are you at risk?

Your health provider can help you determine if you are at risk. You will need to know the following information:

Question	Yes	No
Central obesity. Are you a male with a waist circumference greater than 40 inches or are you female with a waist circumference greater than 35 inches?	❑ Yes	❑ No
Are your fasting triglycerides greater than 150 mg / dl?	❑ Yes	❑ No
Is your HDL less than 40 mg / dl if you are male or less than 50 mg / dl if you are female?	❑ Yes	❑ No
Have you already been diagnosed with high blood pressure or have a BP greater than or equal to 130 / 85?	❑ Yes	❑ No
Is your fasting blood sugar (glucose) greater than or equal to 110 mg / dl?	❑ Yes	❑ No

According to the National Institutes of Health, if you have three out of the previous five conditions you have metabolic syndrome.

If so, you are far from alone. An estimated 47 million Americans have metabolic syndrome. That's about 24 percent or one in four adult Americans. Its incidence increases with age: the older you get, the more common it becomes.

Who is at greatest risk?

Findings from the Third National Health and Nutrition Examination Survey

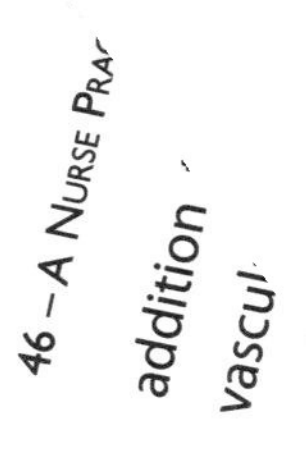

(1988-1994) published in the *Journal of the American*
2002 reported the incidence of metabolic syndrome as

- Mexican Americans had the highest percentaç
- Caucasian Americans (24%) .
- African Americans (22%) .

The same study compared the incidence of metabolic syndrome ...
women and found:

- Among Mexican Americans, women had a 26% higher prevalence than men.
- Among African Americans, women had a 57% higher prevalence than men.
- Among Caucasian Americans, men and women were nearly equally affected.

The tendency toward metabolic syndrome is genetic, but your lifestyle plays a big part in whether or not you ever develop it.

> *If you control your weight, exercise regularly, and eat a healthy diet—even if you have a genetic tendency toward it—you may never develop it. On the other hand, if you become overweight, do not get regular exercise, and eat high-fat foods, you may provoke it.*

Risks associated with metabolic syndrome

It is considered a pre-diabetic state because insulin resistance is part of the syndrome.

Insulin insensitivity is the earliest stage of diabetes. As we just discussed with diabetes, insulin is a hormone made in the pancreas that takes sugar out of the bloodstream and transports it into the cells of the body where it is used for energy. In metabolic syndrome, insulin is present, in fact it may be present at very high levels, but it can't move sugar out of the bloodstream and into the cells. That's because insulin receptors stop working, usually because of the excess weight. For a while the pancreas will make more and more insulin to try to lower the high blood sugar. Eventually, the cells of the pancreas that make the insulin burn out, and that is when full-blown type 2 diabetes develops.

There are other chemical factors present in metabolic syndrome in

...o insulin insensitivity that create conditions that can lead to ... disease and cardiovascular accidents.

...bdominal or central obesity, for example, causes fat to be deposited not ...st in "love handles" but deep in the abdomen where it wraps itself around the internal organs. This deep fat (called *visceral fat*) produces chemicals called *cytokines*. Cytokines are chemical messengers in the body that cause inflammatory responses. Cytokines not only trigger inflammation in blood vessel walls, they also increase the tendency to form blood clots, raise blood pressure, worsen cholesterol profiles, and make insulin resistance worse. The best way to lower the cytokines in your body, and thus all the associated risks, is to lose weight. If you will drop as little as 10 to 15 pounds, you can *significantly* lower the activity of these dangerous chemicals in your body.

This tendency to form blood clots is another danger in metabolic syndrome and why aspirin, a blood thinner, is prescribed for those who have it. If clots break off from the blood vessel walls, they can cause blockages of a coronary artery or a vessel in the brain. That is how some heart attacks and strokes happen.

Metabolic syndrome is more responsive to lifestyle changes than it is to medications, but both are necessary to lower your risks.

Lifestyle changes that reduce risk

Weight loss and exercise (after you have been medically cleared) are the most effective treatments. If you find you have metabolic syndrome, study the sections on Blood Pressure, Cholesterol, Weight and Nutrition, Diabetes, and Cardiovascular Disease. You will see that metabolic syndrome is a collection of all of those conditions. See your healthcare practitioner and agree to aggressive treatment with medications. Make your own personal commitment to change your behaviors. Medications help, but behavior change is the very best treatment. Here's what to do:

- **Lose weight.** Even a loss of 10 to 15 pounds will significantly reduce your risk of diabetes, cardiovascular disease, heart attack, and stroke. If you have metabolic syndrome and are overweight, weight loss is not cosmetic, *it's critical.*

- **Exercise.** Burning up sugar, calories, and fat with exe
you lose weight, prevent diabetes, control blood pressu
cholesterol, and strengthen your heart. In addition, it will
mood and give you the fighting spirit you need to take con
your lifestyle choices. At least 30 minutes of exercise (working
60 minutes) most days of the week is recommended. Exercise wi
increase your HDL and lower your triglycerides. Walking is usually a
safe way to start if you haven't exercised before. You should not begi
a vigorous exercise regimen until your health practitioner has medically cleared you to do so.
- **Eat a healthy, low-fat diet.** You don't have to eat perfectly; you just have to eat better. You want to decrease the fat and calories you consume. Lowering the fat in your diet will help with weight loss and lower your high triglycerides. Watch your portion sizes. Try to eat more unrefined foods like whole grains, fruits, vegetables, and legumes, and get plenty of fiber. Drink lots of water. Cut down on refined foods like sweets, baked goods, and foods with a high glycemic index, which will raise your blood sugar, make you feel hungrier, and make it harder to lose weight. If you have metabolic syndrome, it will help you to learn more about diabetic diets and glycemic control. Understanding how sugars act in your body and blood will help you prevent or control diabetes.
- **Control your blood pressure.** If you have metabolic syndrome, you want your blood pressure to be *less* than 120 / 70. A combination of exercise and weight loss alone may achieve this. If your blood pressure is greater than 120 / 70, see your health practitioner for medication.
- **Control your blood sugar.** If you have elevated fasting blood sugars and insulin insensitivity, do not ignore this warning. Keep an eye on your blood sugars. You may be able to prevent diabetes with lifestyle changes alone, but if your blood sugars start to rise, you need medication. You can check your blood sugars yourself by purchasing a blood sugar monitor for sale at drugstores.
- **Control your cholesterol.** High tryglycerides and low HDL are hallmarks of metabolic syndrome. (That doesn't mean your total cholesterol and LDL aren't high, too, but often they are normal.)

ed to get your cholesterol profile where it ought

is a deadly habit for everyone, but there are oking is particularly deadly: people with ple with lung disease, and people with moke, it is your biggest health risk.

> *ndrome is possibly the messiest and scariest e risks, but it is also the most preventable. Making lifestyle changes and working with your health practitioner can make all the difference.*

High Blood Pressure

An estimated 65 million people (or one in three adults in the United States) have high blood pressure. The medical term for high blood pressure is *hypertension*. A higher percentage of men than women have it before age 55. After age 55, a higher percentage of women than men have it. All cardiovascular diseases, including high blood pressure, develop later in women's lives after the hormonal changes of menopause. After menopause, women's cardiovascular risks are equal to those of men. High blood pressure increases with age in both sexes, from age 55 into the mid-70s. High blood pressure is a particularly dangerous risk for African Americans, whose blood pressures tend to run higher. It's also dangerous in people with diabetes because they often have other vascular disease.

> *The combination of diabetes and high blood pressure increase risks in both conditions. According to the American Diabetes Association, more than 70 percent of people with diabetes also have high blood pressure, and more than 40 percent of them are doing nothing to treat it.*

You will learn that when high blood pressure and cardiovascular disease (CVD) occur together (and they often do in diabetes), the risk of heart attack and stroke as well as other vascular diseases significantly increases. That's why, even if you don't have symptoms, you are wise to know and control your blood pressure.

Are you at risk?

All of us could be. Answering "yes" to any of the following questions means you are at risk.

Question	Yes	No
Is the top number of your BP greater than or equal to 140?	❑ Yes	❑ No
Is the bottom number of your BP above 80?	❑ Yes	❑ No
Have you been diagnosed with high blood pressure or prescribed BP medication?	❑ Yes	❑ No
Do you neglect to take your medication *exactly* as prescribed?	❑ Yes	❑ No
Is your diet high in salt or sodium? (Answer *yes* if you do not know.)	❑ Yes	❑ No
Is your Body Mass Index (BMI) greater than 25?	❑ Yes	❑ No
Do you exercise less than 240 minutes a week at your target heart rate?	❑ Yes	❑ No
Do you smoke?	❑ Yes	❑ No
Are you male and drink more than 24 oz. of beer, 10 oz. of wine, OR 1 oz. of hard liquor per day?	❑ Yes	❑ No
Are you female and drink more than 12 oz. of beer, 5 oz. of wine, OR ½ oz. of hard liquor per day?	❑ Yes	❑ No
Does high blood pressure run in your family?	❑ Yes	❑ No
Are you age 50 or older?	❑ Yes	❑ No
Are you black or African American?	❑ Yes	❑ No

To understand blood pressure, consider a garden hose with the water turned on full blast. If you bend the hose, the pressure builds up inside the hose. The blood pressure in the body works in a similar way. The pumping of blood by the beating heart into the blood vessels of the body is what creates blood pressure. If blood pressure gets too low, the blood can't reach the vital organs and it will lead to death. If blood pressure is too high, its force will damage vital organs by destroying the fragile vessels that deliver blood to the cells.

Blood pressure is gauged by measuring the force of blood against the walls of the blood vessels, both when your heart beats and when your heart rests. The top number of a blood pressure is called the *systolic BP* (SBP). That is the highest pressure in your blood vessels and occurs when your heart beats. The bottom number is called the *diastolic BP* (DBP). That is the lowest pressure in your blood vessels that occurs when your heart rests between heartbeats. Blood pressure is written as SBP / DBP or 120 / 80. It is verbally reported as 120 over 80. The optimal healthy blood pressure reading is less than 120 / 80. Anything under those numbers is considered healthy. Anything over that should be treated with lifestyle changes. Medications should be prescribed if your blood pressure is greater than or equal to 140 / 90, or 130 / 80 if you have diabetes or kidney disease.

High blood pressure is called the silent killer because odds are you won't feel anything. You may never have any symptoms. High blood pressure causes harm because it damages the tiny, fragile end blood vessels that feed the vital target organs. These fragile vessels are not strong enough to withstand the force of the high blood pressure. Vessels in the heart, the brain, the kidneys, the lungs, legs, arms, and retina of the eye are all vulnerable to damage from high blood pressure.

Any blood pressure higher than normal puts you at risk.

If your blood pressure is very high, you are at risk in the short term. If your blood pressure is only a little high but stays a little high for a very long time, you are at risk over the long term.

The long-term risks of high blood pressure include:

- Aneurysm
- Congestive heart failure
- Coronary artery disease
- Enlarged heart (left ventricular hypertrophy = LVH)
- Erectile dysfunction
- Heart attack
- Kidney disease
- Peripheral vascular disease
- Retinopathy (damage to the eyes—can lead to blindness)

- Stroke
- TIA (transient ischemic attack or mini-stroke)

One-third of people who have high blood pressure don't know they have it. According to the American Heart Association, high blood pressure increases your risk of heart attack by 20 percent to 25 percent, your risk of stroke by 35 percent, and your risk of congestive heart failure by 50 percent. *It is the number one preventable risk factor for stroke.*

> *Only 29 percent of people who know they have high blood pressure are on enough medication to adequately control it. Most people need multiple drugs to get blood pressure down to normal, yet many people resist medications mistakenly thinking they are healthier without them. It's the high pressure that's unhealthy and risky, not the drugs that control it.*

If you are diagnosed with high blood pressure, you should be seeing your practitioner until your blood pressure is controlled to less than 140 / 90 if you do not have diabetes or kidney disease, and to less than 130 / 80 if you do. At home, you should be keeping track of your own blood pressure readings and take a written list of them with you each time you see your practitioner. You should take your medications faithfully and exactly as described.

How to accurately monitor your own blood pressure

- **Purchase a blood-pressure machine** or use the ones provided in pharmacies and discount stores.
- **Sit quietly** with your feet on the floor for about 5 minutes before taking your blood pressure to be sure the measurement is accurate.
- **Do not smoke or drink caffeine** for 30 minutes prior to taking your blood pressure.
- **Always write down** the blood pressures you measured, noting the date and time of day you checked it. (Fold a small card in your wallet to use.)
- **Bring all your blood pressure readings** to your health practitioner each time you visit.

- **Tell your doctor or healthcare provider** all medications you are taking including over-the-counter drugs and supplements.

If you have high blood pressure, you must be careful of the over-the-counter medications. Many for sale will increase your blood pressure—possibly to dangerous levels. The most common culprits are cold medications. Aside from some of the newer second-generation antihistamines (like *Claritin*), almost all cold medications should be avoided if you have high blood pressure. Decongestants, while offering nasal symptom relief, elevate blood pressure. Nasal sprays, like *Neosynephrine* and *Afrin*, will also increase blood pressure. Always ask the pharmacist about any over-the-counter medication you plan to take if you have high blood pressure. Other common over-the-counter medications that can raise blood pressure are the anti-inflammatories like *Advil, Motrin,* and *Aleve. Tylenol* and aspirin do not raise blood pressure. If you are taking these other medications, you should monitor your blood pressure closely to make sure they are not raising it above your goal.

High blood pressure is controllable. Proper medication, your healthcare provider's guidance, plus your willingness to make lifestyle changes, can help you bring your blood pressure under control.

The following behaviors help you reach and remain at your goal blood pressure:

- **Exercise.** It lowers blood pressure by increasing the strength of the heart (a muscular pump) and improving the pliability of the blood vessels. The best exercises for lowering blood pressure are rhythmic aerobic activities like walking, biking, swimming, and jogging. These exercises increase the heart rate and use the large muscle groups. They are more effective at lowering blood pressure than lifting weights because they tone the muscular walls of the vascular system. Your blood vessels are small hollow muscles that pump blood. Your heart is a big muscular pump that provides the thrust. Strong and fit muscles in your blood vessels are pliable and toned. They stretch out to receive blood and clamp down to push it with ease. When they are constantly trying to push against high blood pressure, they lose their elasticity and strength and become rigid and weak. Exercise helps your blood vessels get in shape just as it strengthens your heart and other muscles. **Aerobic activities** sustained for 30 to 60 minutes at your target heart rate and performed most days of the week can effectively lower blood pressure. ***Caution:*** If you have not been active, if you have a family history of heart disease, or if you have blood pressure that is greater than or equal to 160 / 90, you should have an exercise stress test before beginning an exercise program. Gentle walking is usually safe, regardless of your exercise history, so long as you do not experience chest pain or abnormal shortness of breath during activity or at rest. See the Exercise chapter to learn more about your target heart rate.

- **Lose weight.** Weight loss lowers blood pressure by decreasing the workload on the heart. Excess weight is like carrying a bag of bricks every day of your life and stresses the heart as well as the joints and spine. When combined with exercise, weight loss is even more effective at lowering blood pressure.
- **Stop smoking.** Smoking interferes in three ways with blood pressure. Remember that the whole point of blood pressure is to pump or circulate oxygen in the blood to the cells of the body.
    - First, smoking causes blood vessels to constrict and that increases blood pressure (like when you bend a garden hose).
    - Second, the poisons in smoke and tobacco products damage the lining of blood vessels (the endothelium).
    - And, last but not least, smoking decreases the amount of oxygen in the blood.
- **Follow the DASH diet.** DASH stands for *Dietary Approaches to Stop Hypertension*. It is a diet rich in fruits, vegetables, and low-fat dairy foods. It is low in saturated fat—the bad fat that comes from animal products like fatty meats that raise cholesterol. It is also low in total fat, sodium, and cholesterol. It is high in dietary fiber, potassium, calcium, and magnesium, and moderately high in protein. You can find books on the DASH diet in bookstores or at the library, or search for Internet sites that cover it in detail and include sample meal plans.

- **Control diabetes.** People who have diabetes are five times more likely to suffer a stroke. If you have diabetes, you want to keep *both* your blood sugars *and* your blood pressure in tight control.
- **Drink alcohol moderately.** Excessive alcohol consumption increases blood pressure. The American Heart Association recommends that if your blood pressure is uncontrolled, you should not drink at all. For those whose blood pressure is controlled and who do not have problems with alcohol abuse, moderate alcohol use (particularly red wine) has been shown to have some health benefits. According to the U.S. Department of Health and Human Services, moderate alcohol consumption is 24 oz. beer, 10 oz. wine, or 2 oz. 100-proof whiskey per day for men, half that amount for women.
- **Reduce salt.** Sodium (or salt) draws water into the blood vessels. It increases the circulating blood volume and, as a result, increases blood pressure. Limit the salt (sodium) in your diet to less than 2,300 mg per day. You can find sodium content on all food labels, and when you do, don't forget to bear in mind the serving size of the food in question. Processed foods tend to have high sodium levels, especially canned soups, tomato-based products, smoked meats, crackers, and chips. As an ethnic group, African Americans are particularly sensitive to sodium and can sometimes lower blood pressure by simply restricting sodium in their diet. Usually, though, medication is also required.
- **Practice relaxation techniques.** Biofeedback is a technique by which you can learn to gain voluntary control over physiological processes like your heart rate, amount of muscle tension, and blood pressure. Meditation is another method that teaches you how to relax. With practice, these techniques can slow the heart and lower blood pressure by conditioning a relaxation response that you can call upon whenever you need it.

All the changes above can make a remarkable difference in the prevention and treatment of high blood pressure. Choose one, choose two, and ***make the change.***

High Cholesterol

According to the American Heart Association, more than 100 million American adults have total cholesterol levels greater than 200 mg / dL. High cholesterol (called *hypercholesterolemia* or *hyperlipidemia*) is a major risk factor for cardiovascular disease. Cholesterol is a fatty substance produced mostly in the liver and, to a lesser degree, in other body tissues. It is also present in certain foods, although only a small amount of our cholesterol comes from food (our bodies make most of it). The liver produces cholesterol to help absorb fat. That's why a high-fat diet increases cholesterol. Cholesterol also goes into making vitamin D and various steroid hormones like estrogen, testosterone, and cortisol. Cholesterol can sometimes crystallize in the gallbladder and form gallstones.

Imagine that a thick and sticky sludge is flowing through your blood vessels. Over many years, it sticks to the walls of the vessels and clogs them up resulting in decreased blood flow through the vessels. When cholesterol combines with LDL (a lipoprotein that carries cholesterol throughout the body), it worms its way inside the lining of blood vessel walls. These cholesterol deposits are called plaques and they can break through or rupture into the vessel's opening. When that happens in the coronary arteries or vessels in the brain, it causes heart attack or stroke.

Are you at risk?

To know if you are at risk from high cholesterol, you need a blood test called a cholesterol (or lipid) profile ordered for you by your health practitioner. When you know the results of the blood test, you and your healthcare practitioner can answer these questions to determine if you are at risk.

Is your total cholesterol *greater* than 200 mg / dl?	❑ Yes	❑ No
Are your triglycerides *greater* than 150 mg / dl? (See the metabolic syndrome chapter.)	❑ Yes	❑ No

Question	Yes	No
Is your HDL (good) cholesterol *less* than 40 mg / dl? (If your HDL is *greater* than 60 mg / dl your risk from high cholesterol is lowered!)	❑ Yes	❑ No
Is your LDL (bad) cholesterol *greater* than 100 mg / dl?	❑ Yes	❑ No
Is your blood pressure *greater than* or *equal to* 140 / 90 (130 / 80 if you have diabetes or metabolic syndrome)?	❑ Yes	❑ No
Do you eat a diet high in fat and cholesterol?	❑ Yes	❑ No
Do you smoke?	❑ Yes	❑ No
Do you exercise less than 240 minutes per week at your target heart rate?	❑ Yes	❑ No
Is your Body Mass Index (BMI) greater than 25?	❑ Yes	❑ No
Do you have any forms of cardiovascular disease (CVD):		
• Coronary artery disease?	❑ Yes	❑ No
• Carotid artery disease?	❑ Yes	❑ No
• Peripheral vascular disease?	❑ Yes	❑ No
• Renal artery disease?	❑ Yes	❑ No
• Abdominal aortic aneurysm?	❑ Yes	❑ No
Do you have metabolic syndrome or diabetes?	❑ Yes	❑ No
Do you have a family history of high cholesterol?	❑ Yes	❑ No
Do you have a family history of heart disease or stroke?	❑ Yes	❑ No

If you answered yes to one or more of these questions, read on. You are at risk.

The process of high cholesterol began in our teen years, helped along by all the burgers and pizza we ate. The buildup of fatty, cholesterol deposits in the blood vessels is called either arteriosclerosis or atherosclerosis; both mean the same thing. These deposits eventually get hard and turn into what are called plaques. Over time either the space inside the vessels gets smaller from the buildup (as in a clogged drain pipe) or plaque that's built up inside the vessel wall grows large enough to rupture or break through and cause a blockage.

If the plaque builds up gradually along the lining of the blood vessel (which is like a hose), the opening gets smaller and the pressure inside the hose goes up; this can cause high blood pressure.

If the plaque ruptures into a vessel's opening (or lumen) and blocks it, the supply of blood will be cut off to the area that the blood vessel feeds. That results in the death of those cells that no longer get any blood. If the arteries of the heart get blocked, the result is a heart attack. If vessels in the brain get blocked, the result is a stroke or brain attack.

Risks of cholesterol buildup

- **Coronary heart disease or blockages** in the coronary arteries without heart attack.
- **Arteriosclerosis or atherosclerosis** (blockages in vessels anywhere in the body—heart, brain, kidneys, legs, eyes, fingers, toes, etc.)
- **Carotid artery disease**—a blockage of one or both of the large carotid arteries that are on both sides of the neck and supply blood to the brain.
- **Renal artery disease**—a narrowing or blockage of the large arteries that pump blood through the kidneys.
- **Peripheral vascular disease**—blockages in the vessels of the legs or arms.

If you already know you have any form of cardiovascular disease (CVD) or a risk equivalent such as diabetes or metabolic syndrome and you have high cholesterol, you should be on medication.

> *Many people are unable to reach target cholesterol levels with lifestyle changes alone. It may be your genes rather than your lifestyle that are causing your high cholesterol.*

In that case, you will need medication *and* lifestyle changes to reach your goal. Remember, getting to goal numbers, not avoiding medication, is what will lower your risks from high cholesterol.

Cholesterol medications have been controversial. They are expensive and require regular blood tests to check liver function. According to a joint report by the National Heart, Lung, and Blood Institute; American College of Cardiology Foundation; and American Heart Association, *these medications are under-prescribed and are safe for the overwhelming majority of people who need them.* Clinical trials so far show that they significantly decrease the risk of heart attack and stroke and reduce peripheral vascular disease. In addition to lowering cholesterol, the medications also seem to stabilize plaque and decrease inflammation in the vessels, thus reducing the incidence of plaque rupture that leads to heart attack and stroke.

If you need cholesterol medication, you will probably need to be on it for life. If you reach target numbers with medication and then stop taking it, your cholesterol numbers will likely rise again. Based on what we know today, uncontrolled high cholesterol is much more dangerous than the drugs used to lower it. Whether cholesterol medication is right for you is something you need to discuss with your health practitioner.

It is your responsibility to do everything within your power to take control of this risk. Exercise, weight loss, and a healthy diet may be all you need to do to manage this risk before it gets dangerously out of hand. Until you know your cholesterol profile you can not begin to handle this risk. It is in your best interest to get a blood test and learn what your cholesterol profile is.

An optimal cholesterol profile looks like this:

- **Total cholesterol is less than 200.**
- **LDL (low-density lipoproteins) is less than 130 mg / dl if you have no other risks; less than 100 mg / dl if you have known cardiovascular disease, diabetes, or metabolic syndrome.** This is the bad cholesterol. It works its way into blood vessel walls and causes damage (this is called soft plaque). It also builds up along the lining of the vessel walls and causes blockages (this is called hard plaque). Both types of plaque can rupture and cause heart attacks and strokes (brain attacks). LDL comes in three sizes—all are bad. The smallest LDL is thought to be the most dangerous. Small LDL particles penetrate the artery walls more easily than large LDLs and become trapped there. Their cholesterol is released and this causes plaque to build up.
- **HDL (high-density lipoproteins) is greater than 50 mg / dl in men and greater than 55 mg / dl in women.** This is the good cholesterol because of its high density. It rolls through your blood vessels like a bowling ball knocking bad plaque off the vessel walls and cleaning out the vessels. Large HDL particles remove cholesterol from the arteries, while small HDL do not. Because of this action, HDL actually

improves the health of your blood vessels. That's why having levels of HDL greater than 60 mg / dl is protective.

- **Triglycerides are less than 150 mg / dl.** These are fats that circulate around in your blood, and they also increase your heart attack or stroke risk.
- **VLDL (very low density lipoproteins) is less than 30 mg / dl.** This is the very bad cholesterol. VLDL works its way easily inside the vessel walls to cause plaque. Large VLDL particles are the most dangerous and are most affected by how much fat you eat. High levels are associated with increased risk of arteriosclerosis and heart attack and stroke. They are a subset (or type) of LDL.

Currently, treatment for high cholesterol is based mostly on the cholesterol profile outlined above along with consideration for your other risk factors. As there are many variations in cholesterol profiles, the significance of your particular cholesterol and risk profile should be discussed with your health practitioner.

The goals or targets for cholesterol treatment continue to evolve. These guidelines are endorsed by the National Heart, Lung, and Blood Institute; American College of Cardiology Foundation; and American Heart Association, and are current at the time of this writing. Cholesterol goals or targets are revised periodically based on ongoing research, and they keep getting lowered. Experts aren't sure how low cholesterol should be, but at present they believe the lower the better for everyone—regardless of other risks.

If you have less than two of the risk factors listed at the beginning of the chapter and have just discovered your cholesterol is elevated, a 12-week trial of lifestyle changes is a reasonable approach to see if you can reach target numbers without medication.

Here's how you can reduce your cholesterol levels without medication:

- **Exercise.** It will burn up fat and cholesterol and increase the metabolic rate at which your body uses energy and burns up calories. People who exercise burn more fat and calories even at rest than people who are sedentary. Since cholesterol is a fat, increasing the metabolic rate will lower cholesterol levels.

- **Lose weight.** This is especially important if your body mass index (BMI) is higher than 25. BMI is a formula that uses weight and height to estimate body fat and gauge health risks because of carrying too much weight. Being overweight and having high cholesterol often go together. Weight loss often results in an improved cholesterol profile.
- **Follow a low-fat, low-cholesterol diet.** Foods that are high in cholesterol are all of animal origin. Examples are fatty cuts of meat, the skin of chicken, egg yolk, butter, cream, whole milk, cheese, and baked goods made with butter. To lower the cholesterol in your diet, switch to lean meats and skinless chicken; limit egg yolks, butter, and cream; switch to low-fat milk; substitute frozen yogurt for ice cream; and decrease baked sweets.
- **Quit smoking.** Smoking and high cholesterol are related by chemical reactions that occur inside the blood vessels. Smoking introduces chemicals into the bloodstream that cause the cholesterol plaques in the vessels to become unstable. Smoking also inflames the lining of the blood vessels and makes it easier for plaque to break off. At the same time smoking constricts the vessels. The combination of these effects results in a much higher risk that pieces of plaque will break off and cause obstruction of a blood vessel, resulting in a heart attack, a stroke (brain attack), or a blood clot somewhere else in the body.

High cholesterol is manageable, but it does require attention. Together you and your healthcare provider can bring the numbers to target. And then, it's just a matter of keeping them there.

Depression

Depression is a mental illness. It is not a bad mood, poor outlook, or inability to cope.

Everyone experiences depressed thoughts or feelings at some time, but it is important to distinguish a passing mood or a temporary response to difficult circumstances from the disease known as depression.

Depression not only involves emotions and thoughts, but it affects one's most basic bodily functions, too. It affects how a person eats, sleeps, thinks, and acts. It is not the result of personal weakness. It cannot be willed or wished away. A person doesn't "just get over it" without help and treatment.

Many people who suffer from depression or know family members or friends who are suffering from depression, don't realize that depression is a medical disorder with chemical and biological causes. Understand that depression is highly treatable. Don't be like millions of Americans who suffer, not realizing they have a treatable disease.

According to the National Institute of Mental Health, approximately 21 million American adults or almost 10 percent of the United States' population has a depressive disorder. One in five people will be affected by depression at some point in life. Nearly twice as many women as men are affected by a depression. Major depressive disorder is the number one cause of disability for those 15 to 44 years of age.

Are you at risk?

Question	Yes	No
Do you have persistent depressed, sad, anxious, or empty moods?	❑ Yes	❑ No
Do you feel worthless, helpless, or guilty?	❑ Yes	❑ No
Do you feel hopeless about the future?	❑ Yes	❑ No
Are you overly pessimistic?	❑ Yes	❑ No
Have you lost interest or pleasure in your usual activities?	❑ Yes	❑ No
Are you suffering decreased energy and feel chronic fatigue?	❑ Yes	❑ No
Do you have difficulties with your memory, concentration, or decision making?	❑ Yes	❑ No
Do you have increased irritability, restlessness, or agitation?	❑ Yes	❑ No
Do you sleep either too much or too little?	❑ Yes	❑ No
Have you had a loss of appetite or are you overeating in response to your emotional state?	❑ Yes	❑ No

Do you have recurring thoughts of death or suicide?	❑ Yes	❑ No
Are you an alcoholic or drug addict?	❑ Yes	❑ No
Have you suffered a recent loss?	❑ Yes	❑ No
Do you suffer from a chronic illness?	❑ Yes	❑ No
Do you have a family history of depression?	❑ Yes	❑ No

If you answered yes to any of the statements and you have experienced them for ***longer than two weeks,*** *you are at risk for depression.*

Our brains are complex organs and control all that we think and feel. The chemistry of the brain is a major contributor to its function. Chemicals in the brain influence our moods, thoughts, and behaviors. These chemicals are called *neurotransmitters.*

How brain chemistry works

The brain is made up of millions and millions of nerve cells called neurons. These neurons communicate with one another by sending chemical signals across small spaces in between the cells. These spaces are known as *synapses.* Imagine two dominos lying side by side with a small space in between them. The dominos represent the neurons and the space represents the synapse. One neuron releases chemicals into that space and the neurotransmitters (the chemical signals) are either picked up and taken inside the neuron on the other side of the space, or they are blocked. Neurotransmitters have different effects depending on the particular chemical, how much of it is released, and how much the next cell either takes up and absorbs or blocks. This is a very complicated chemical event, and an abnormality in this brain chemistry is believed to cause many forms of depression. The medications we use to treat depression correct the chemical imbalance and normalize the chemistry in the brain.

These three main neurotransmitters are known, and more are being studied:

- **Serotonin** is a neurotransmitter that influences learning, sleep, and control of mood. Long-term stress will tend to lower serotonin levels and cause depression, problems with concentration, and memory.

- **Norepinephrine** influences alertness. Imbalances of norepinephrine may result in lethargic feelings or lack of energy. Low levels also contribute to depression and memory problems. Too much will cause the opposite: being hyper-alert and overly excited.
- **Dopamine** is involved in pleasure sensations, cognition, mental capacity, motivation, attention, as well as movement and motor function. Imbalances in dopamine are believed to influence other mental conditions in addition to depression, like Parkinson's disease and schizophrenia.

As we begin to understand what these chemicals do, it is easy to see how abnormal levels can create problems with mood, psychological capacities, and feelings. Abnormalities in this chemistry interfere with one's ability to work and interact with the world.

Family history and genetic predisposition

Brain chemistry isn't the only thing that causes depression —family history and genetics also play a role.

Although a direct genetic link has not yet been discovered, as many as 80 percent to 90 percent of people with depression have family members who also have suffered from depression. Although you might inherit a risk of developing depression, you may never develop the disease unless some difficult life circumstance provokes it.

There are three types of depression:

- **Dysthymia.** This is having long-term sad and pessimistic feelings that keep you from functioning or feeling well. You just feel bad and sad all the time. This disorder lasts two years or longer and is less disabling than major depression. While it is not disabling, if you suffer from dysthymia, you are at increased risk of experiencing a major depressive episode at some time in your life. Three-quarters of those who suffer dysthymia have some other psychiatric or medical disorder. If left untreated, dysthymia may lead to major depression, alcoholism, or suicide.
- **Major depression.** This is a combination of symptoms that includes emotional, mental, and physical disturbances. Major depression

interferes with your ability to work, study, sleep, eat, and enjoy activities you once found pleasurable. If you have been experiencing symptoms for longer than two weeks, you may be suffering depression. You will benefit from seeing your health practitioner or a mental healthcare professional to receive treatment. Major depression may only occur once in your life, but more commonly it occurs several times over the course of a lifetime. Receiving treatment may decrease its occurrence and lessen its impact on your life.

- **Bipolar disorder (also known as manic-depressive disorder).** This is a less common form of depression characterized by mood swings. According to the National Institute of Mental Health, almost 6 million American adults suffer bipolar disorder in any given year. The disorder is characterized by euphoric high moods (mania) that alternate with very low and hopeless moods (depression). In some people, the mood swings are rapid and dramatic, but in most they are gradual. A person in a manic phase may make poor choices and suffer professional, personal, or romantic embarrassment. Mania that is not treated can progress to a psychotic state where the person actually loses touch with reality. Like diabetes or heart disease, bipolar disorder is a long-term illness that must be carefully managed throughout a person's life.

  There are three types of bipolar disorder.

  - In *bipolar I*, a person has experienced a full-blown episode of mania and also suffers from periods of depression.
  - *Bipolar II* is similar but less extreme.
  - *Bipolar III* refers to a person who has only experienced depressive states, no mania, but has a strong family history of bipolar disorder. Also, people who develop mania when they are treated with certain anti-depressants, plus have a family history of bipolar disorder are considered type III.

Alcohol and drug abuse are very common among people with bipolar disorder. But when their illness is properly treated, people with bipolar disorder can lead healthy and productive lives. It is important that medications be taken without fail. When people with bipolar disorder stop taking their medications the illness can spiral out of control. If this happens, hospitalization for p stabilization may be necessary to correct the chemical imba that result from not taking medication properly.

Any form of depression that goes untreated will undermine all your oth efforts at risk reduction. Its characteristic sadness and hopelessness can lead to a host of unhealthy behaviors that will interfere with your ability to carry out the plans and goals you make for yourself. The biggest risk of depression is not treating it.

Nearly 74 percent of Americans who seek help for depression go to a primary health practitioner rather than a mental health professional. Many will consult health practitioners thinking they have a physical illness when, in fact, they are actually suffering from depression. This is called *masked depression*. In masked depression physical symptoms are not recognized as being caused by depression.

The diagnosis of depression is missed half of the time by health practitioners in primary care settings.

You must be open, honest, and clear with your practitioner so that they may help you in the necessary and appropriate manner. If you feel depressed or can claim any of the previous risk questions as true, it is your responsibility to share that information with your practitioner who is there to help you. Seek care if you are depressed and don't be afraid to say you are depressed.

Major depressive disorders are replacing stroke as the leading cause of disability in the United States. The World Health Organization estimates that by the year 2020, major depression will be second only to chronic heart disease as an international health burden. Yet, according to the National Institute of Mental Health, more than 50 percent of those suffering depression either never seek help or never receive treatment.

Remember that ***depression is treatable.***

More than 80 percent of people with depression can be treated successfully with medication, psychotherapy, or a combination of both. There is no shame in needing help, or in getting it. With treatment, depression will lift and you will regain your sense of purpose and drive. A full, healthy, and happy life awaits. Seek help if you need it.

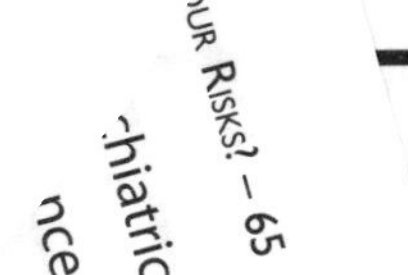

Stress and Anxiety

stress is universal. Everyone experiences it at some eadline at work or a first date, life's challenges and stress. Some people live very high stress lives and some low, but everyone experiences stress at one time or another.

Anxiety disorders differ from stress in that they last for at least six months. Those with anxiety disorder live with constant worrisome thoughts about everyday life. They always think that the worst will happen even when there is little reason to expect it. Anxiety and depression commonly occur together.

Like depression, both of these conditions are treatable. Anxiety disorders are the most common mental illness in America, surpassing even depression in numbers. According to the National Institute of Mental Health, approximately 40 million adults in the United States suffer anxiety disorders. It is the most common mental health problem in elders over 65 years of age. Women suffer from anxiety and stress almost twice as much as men. Workplace stress has come under increased scrutiny in recent years as a problem that is bad for both employees and businesses.

Stress and anxiety can be thought of on a continuum, with everyday stress on one end and the severe, crippling terror of panic attacks on the opposite end. Stress is a normal part of human life. And it is not always the demon we have grown to believe it to be. Stress is necessary for survival. It heightens the senses and increases alertness. For that reason, stress is protective.

Stress also can be stimulating and lead to growth and achievements. For example, the stress of competition in sports can lead to heightened human performance, like setting new world records. Many a champion has credited top performance to the stress of the competition and the pressure from a worthy opponent or the time clock. The events that happen to you and the way you react to them determine the level of stress you experience.

It is only when stress overwhelms us or impairs our ability to function that it becomes a health problem and a risk factor for disease. How each of us responds to stress depends on our personality type and our life experiences. In general, "good stress" exhilarates; "bad stress" exhausts.

Stress and anxiety can increase your health risks only if they are unmanageable in your life, or if they interfere with your ability to function in a way you would prefer.

Types of Stress

- **Acute stress** is the common, everyday stress we all feel at times. You feel it when someone cuts you off in traffic, if your boss criticizes you, or when you have a fight with your spouse.

  Certain people tend to be more susceptible to stressful reactions. Some people are chronic worriers. They feel their life is always out of control. Also, people who have strong competitive drives often feel stressed. People who tend to feel impatient, experience frequent hostile feelings, and have a sense of urgency about time are more susceptible to stress. More relaxed personalities, or people who take things more easily, are not as troubled by stress as their competitive counterparts. Neither type of personality is good or bad; people just tend to react in different ways under certain circumstances. Understanding your personality type can help you keep things in perspective.

  If you find your automatic gut reactions to things are adding to the stress in your life, there are things you can do to control them. Learning to modify your reactions and thoughts about the things that stress you can change your whole outlook and greatly reduce the stress you feel. *Acute stress is a highly **self-treatable** condition.*
- **Chronic stress** is the kind of stress that doesn't go away. It is relentless. It wears you down day after day, year after year. Life circumstances such as dysfunctional families, unhappy marriages, despised jobs, poverty, ethnic conflict (like that currently in Iraq, Afghanistan, and the rest of the Middle East, and areas of Northern Ireland, for example) can result in unending stress for individuals.

  Long-term behavioral and / or medical treatments, aided by a strong personal desire to rise above these ashes of despair, can defeat this type of stress. Those who survive and are able to prevail over chronic stress may ultimately find peace and happiness. There are countless stories of individuals who survived horrifying life experiences and went on to build happy lives, accomplish remarkable achievements, and find personal peace and contentment.

Both types of stress can lead to a host of health problems.

Some of the risks include:

- Asthma
- Cancer
- Chest pains
- Chronic fatigue
- Colitis
- Coronary artery disease
- Depression
- Diabetes
- Eating disorders
- Eczema
- Gastric ulcers
- Headaches
- Heart attack
- High blood pressure
- Insomnia
- Irritable bowel syndrome
- Lung disease
- Memory problems
- Muscular pain and tension
- Obesity
- Palpitations
- Poor concentration
- Sexual dysfunction
- Stomach upset
- Stroke
- Substance abuse (drugs and / or alcohol)
- Suicide
- Violence
- Weakened immunity

Living with frequent acute stress reactions and finding it difficult to relax, or suffering chronic stress for which there is no perceived escape, can progress into an *anxiety disorder*. Phobias, obsessive compulsive disorder, or panic disorder are psychiatric conditions that require treatment. Anxiety disorders differ from acute stress in that they last longer than two weeks. They are also often accompanied by physical symptoms like fatigue, nausea, bowel disorders, headaches, or muscle tension.

If you find yourself living in a state of chronic stress or suffering an anxiety disorder, you are at risk of reaching a state of exhaustion in which both your physical and mental health are vulnerable to breakdown. People under constant stress have weaker immune systems and are more prone to all forms of illness. The constant barrage of stress hormones may also increase your risk of cardiovascular accidents like heart attack and stroke, or even sudden death from an acute stress reaction.

This acute stress reaction is an evolutionary necessity that protects us. When facing danger, our fight or flight response causes physical changes in our body that prepare us to either fight or flee. This stress response is an instinctual response to threat. When it is triggered, certain things happen in the body. Chemicals are released in the brain that cause the heart rate to accelerate, the blood pressure to go up, the respiratory rate to increase, the pupils of the eyes to dilate, and the palms to sweat. Blood is quickly shunted away from areas like the gut to the vital organs and the skeletal muscles. There is a release of sugar into the blood, along with other chemicals like cortisol, the stress hormone. It is common to feel emotions like dread, fear, and a sense of impending doom.

These responses are very helpful when faced with a life-threatening danger (like a mugger or a saber-toothed tiger). The problem is that the dangers for which the fight or flight response evolved are uncommon in modern life. If you find you are reacting regularly to daily hassles and undeserved slights with a fight-or-flight response, the constant overload on your system will take its toll over time.

There will be times when you feel anxious. It is just the nature of living. Those who cannot find a healthful outlet for their stress not only risk their physical health, but also put themselves at risk for unhealthy coping behaviors, like addiction.

Those who can learn to deal with these threats in a focused and effective way will cultivate an emotional hardiness. One's resilience grows and future stressors can be managed with more confidence and courage. Turning one's stressors into strengths is one of life's greatest and most rewarding challenges. Believe in yourself. Create the life you desire.

Alcohol and Tobacco

In this section, we are going to talk about alcohol and tobacco, but any addictive behavior will undermine your ability to take control of your health risks. Many substances and behaviors besides alcohol and tobacco can be addictive. Both illegal and legal drugs, food, caffeine, sugar, shopping, sex, pornography, gambling, television, even Internet surfing can become compulsions. In short, any behavior you are compelled to continue even when you would like to stop can be considered an addiction.

The most sensible thing we can do is recognize the risks our compulsions create and try to substitute healthier behaviors for our less healthy ones. Moderation is a way to maintain balance. A rich inner life and cultivating mental resilience will help us find our way to the ecstasy and bliss we seek without destroying our health and our lives.

Alcohol

Alcohol is the most widely used and abused drug in America. Alcohol used by adults in small amounts is considered safe, even beneficial. Therefore, alcohol may or may not be a risk factor in your life. It is when you begin to require alcohol as a coping mechanism that you should seriously examine your alcohol consumption.

Alcohol is a depressant that is made from grapes, grains, and berries and fermented or distilled into a liquid. Alcoholic beverages include beer, wine, and spirits. Because alcohol helps people relax and let down their inhibitions, some people become dependent on it to help them with social anxiety. Alcohol can cause some people to become aggressive. Because most addictive substances require larger and larger amounts to achieve the same effect, their use can easily get out of hand.

Alcohol affects every part of the body. It is carried through the bloodstream to the brain, stomach, muscles, and internal organs including the liver and kidneys. It is absorbed very quickly, in as little as 5 to 10 minutes, and can stay in the body for several hours. Alcohol acts on the central nervous system and slows down brain activity. Over time, heavy drinking causes brain damage. Alcohol poisoning occurs when a person drinks a large quantity of alcohol in a short amount of time (called *binge drinking*). This can be fatal.

Although alcohol abuse often starts early in life, anyone at any age can have a drinking problem. Teenagers who start drinking before age 21 are at higher risk for alcoholism. Seniors who are widowed or retired, who are lonely or suffer health problems and start to drink for comfort are also at risk. The sooner a person realizes that they are abusing alcohol, the better the chances of recovery.

Alcohol use and abuse can be classified into three categories:

- **Alcohol consumption without abuse.**
- **Alcohol abuse**—drinking too much, too often, but without physical or psychological dependence.
- **Alcohol dependence (or alcoholism)**—uncontrolled drinking that interferes with one's occupation, social life, or health and results in physiological and psychological withdrawal symptoms if alcohol consumption is stopped.

There are health risks associated with both alcohol abuse and dependence.

Are you at risk?

To assess your risk, answer each of the following questions honestly with a yes or no.

I feel the need to **Cut down** on my drinking.	❑ Yes	❑ No
I am **Annoyed** if I am criticized about my drinking.	❑ Yes	❑ No
I feel **Guilty** about my drinking.	❑ Yes	❑ No
I sometimes have a drink to get me started (an "**Eye-opener**").	❑ Yes	❑ No

from Ewing JA. Detecting alcoholism, the CAGE questionnaire. JAMA 1984; 252: 1905-1907

If you answered yes to two or more of these questions, you may have a problem with alcohol abuse or dependence.

Few people are able to recover from alcohol dependence without treatment. With treatment, many are able to stop drinking and recover their lives.

Alcohol abuse and dependence are huge health and life risks. Many alcoholics lose everything—jobs, families, money, self-respect—before they seek help. According to the U.S. Department of Health and Human Services, 121 million Americans age 12 and older drink alcohol. Nearly 17 million Americans—1 in every 13 adults—abuse alcohol or are alcoholic. More than one-half of people in the United States report that one or more of their close relatives has a drinking problem.

Different parts of the world propose different safe amounts of alcohol consumption for men and women. Moderate alcohol consumption, according to the U.S. Department of Health Dietary Guidelines for Americans, is the following:

Alcohol "Safe" Limits per Day	Men	Women
Beer	24 oz.	12 oz.
Wine	10 oz.	5 oz.
Hard Liquor	1 oz.	½ oz.

Women's safe amounts are smaller than men's because of their smaller body size and different metabolisms. In addition, every individual has his or her own unique physical and genetic susceptibilities to alcohol. Health complications like alcoholism or liver disease may result from any alcohol consumption at all.

If you drink more than recommended amounts of alcohol, you are at risk. The best way to handle this risk, as with any other, is by being aware of the potential danger. Be alert to your drinking behaviors. Be honest with yourself about who is in control—you or the alcohol. Recognize that an addiction to alcohol can be the first step to serious health risks, not only from the drug itself, but from its contribution to poor decision-making.

Heavy drinkers are frequently heavy smokers, too. Among heavy alcohol users, 60 percent smoke cigarettes. Unlike alcohol, there are no "safe" guidelines for tobacco consumption.

Smoking

Smoking is a life-threatening addiction. Cigarettes, cigars, and snuff are poison-delivery systems—simple as that. Tobacco in any form *significantly* increases your risks of serious chronic and acute diseases. As of this writing, it is the *number one preventable cause of death.* Smoking is the most deadly form of tobacco use, but smokeless tobacco (like chewing and snuff) is also hazardous.

According to the American Heart Association, 48 million American adults smoke. That is 22 percent of American adults over 18 years of age. Smoking has been on the decline among all age groups—*except* young adults. In the age group between 18 and 24 years of age, smoking is actually *increasing.* Five thousand children and adolescents under the age of 18 start smoking every day. Most of them continue to smoke on through adulthood.

Smoking is expected to cause 10 million deaths every year by 2030. One-third of all smokers die prematurely because of their dependence on tobacco. Smokers die 13 to 14 years earlier than non-smokers. According to the CDC, smoking causes more than 438,000 pre-mature deaths (or one in every five deaths) every year. According to the National Cancer Institute, smoking causes one-third of all cancer deaths every year.

Scientists have identified more than 4,800 chemical compounds present in tobacco smoke; so far, 69 of these have been proven to cause cancer in humans and animals. Smoking can cause disease in almost every organ in the body at any age. Wherever blood flows, the cancer-causing chemicals in tobacco go, too.

> *Exposure to secondhand smoke causes an estimated 3,000 nonsmoking adults to die of lung cancer each year. More than 300,000 children suffer lower respiratory tract infections each year because of their exposure to secondhand smoke.*

If you have used tobacco for many years, smoking cessation cannot completely eliminate the risk of developing lung cancer. *But those people who stop smoking by middle age lower their lung cancer risk by more than 90 percent.* If you already have lung disease, it stops getting worse and even starts to improve the minute you stop smoking. But don't be fooled into believing that smoking only causes lung cancer. It comes with a long list of other hazards, too.

Here are just some of the risks of smoking:

Hidden risks

- Abdominal aortic aneurysms
- Cataracts
- Chronic lung disease—emphysema, chronic bronchitis, asthma, COPD (chronic obstructive pulmonary disease), pneumonia
- Diabetes
- Duodenal ulcers, Crohn's disease, and colon polyps
- Gastrointestinal disorders
- Gum disease
- Harm to unborn children of mothers who smoke
- Hearing loss
- Heart disease (twice the risk of non-smokers)
- High blood pressure
- Impotence / erectile dysfunction
- Macular degeneration
- Rheumatoid arthritis
- Stroke

Cancer risks

- Bladder cancer
- Breast cancer
- Cervical cancer
- Colorectal cancer
- Esophageal cancer
- Head and neck cancer
- Kidney cancer
- Leukemia
- Lung cancer
- Stomach cancer
- Mouth or oral cancer
- Pancreatic cancer
- Throat cancer (of the pharynx and larynx)

Treating the diseases caused by smoking costs 75 billion dollars a year, and that doesn't take into account loss of income and productivity from being sick.

If you are lucky enough to consider yourself healthy and you smoke, you can prevent a long list of health problems if you quit now. If you already suffer from chronic diseases like emphysema or cardiovascular disease, your health will begin to improve within days after putting tobacco down. Your risk of heart attack and stroke drops significantly and quickly after quitting.

It seems that everybody who smokes knows they should quit. They also know that quitting tobacco is *hard*. Experts say it is harder to stop smoking than it is to get off heroin or cocaine. Most people try to quit two or three times before they are permanently successful. In spite of that, according to the Surgeon General, 46 million Americans have successfully quit for good.

Most of them will tell you that life really is better without tobacco.

Before the advent of nicotine replacement and medication, people stopped smoking with nothing more than their own desire and determination—and maybe a handful of self-help books. Many of these individuals quit for good. The resources available to you today are much better, and your chances of success are better too.

> *The fundamental battle, however, is unchanged. Nothing can make it easy to stop smoking. If it were easy, everyone would achieve it. You must do battle with the inner demons of addiction to successfully quit smoking for good.*

How hard is it to stop?

You should expect to experience withdrawal symptoms, both physical and psychological. It is normal to fear failure. You may hear self-defeating voices in your head telling you, "I can't do it." You may look around at smokers and think that they, unlike you, are "free" to smoke. That's a trick the addicted brain plays on you. Those smokers aren't "free" to smoke; rather, *you* are "free" *not* to smoke. Smokers are hooked. They wish that they, like you, were strong enough not to smoke.

You may feel a lack of support from friends or family if they continue to smoke or discourage you in your efforts to quit. You may even experience temporary depression or suffer a grief reaction at giving up something you enjoy and that comforts you. That's a normal response. Recognize it as just part of the addiction and what makes quitting so hard.

> *But if quitting smoking is what you truly desire, you will get through it. If you have a strong will to stop—a fire of determination in your belly—you will prevail. It's just a habit. It is entirely possible to create new and healthier habits. Plus, it's a great feeling to be free of the cravings for tobacco. It's worth quite a bit of struggle to achieve that freedom. There are few actions in your life that will make you feel as strong and personally powerful as quitting smoking. Go for it!*

Smoking vs. weight gain

Many people say they would try to quit smoking if they knew they wouldn't gain weight. While it is true most people do gain a little weight when they stop smoking, usually the gain is small (around 5 to 10 pounds) and occurs gradually over several months after quitting.

That minor weight gain in comparison to the health risks posed by smoking is insignificant. The average smoker would have to gain over 75 to 100 pounds to put the additional workload on the heart that is created by smoking, and this doesn't even take into account the cancer risk.

> *It is entirely possible to quit smoking without gaining weight.*

Weight is gained because quitters tend to take in more calories from food for a couple of reasons. Nicotine is an appetite suppressant and so you may feel more hungry in the first weeks after you quit. The absence of cigarettes in your hands and in your mouth may lead you to satisfy cravings for oral stimulation by taking in more food.

However, there are many low-calorie ways to provide oral stimulation. Gum, toothpicks, hard candies, water, fruits, and vegetables can all satisfy oral cravings without adding significant calories. Exercise is a great way to fight cravings, control weight, and improve your overall health. By walking or running you not only prevent weight gain but also enjoy an activity less appreciated by smokers: breathing! Usually, once the non-smoking behavior becomes firmly established, your normal eating patterns will return. At that point, it's not too hard to take off the few pounds you have gained.

If you quit smoking and control your weight, there are more cosmetic benefits you will gain. Non-smokers have fewer wrinkles, better skin, reduced hair loss, improved appearance of their teeth and nails, and a more youthful appearance than smokers do.

If you suffer a relapse, don't despair. Just regroup your resources, review your reasons for quitting, give yourself credit for trying, and start planning for your next quit date.

Change—a sneak preview [1]

Managing and sustaining a behavioral change like quitting smoking takes time and commitment. Your chances of success will improve if you line up support and recognize from the beginning that there will be setbacks. Getting support and anticipating setbacks is just good planning.

> *Always remember that two steps forward, one step back is still progress that moves you forward.*

It is natural to feel discouraged by a setback, but don't lose sight of the progress you are making or abandon your goal. It's the big picture and the long-term outcome you want to keep clear in your mind. Do not be distracted or led astray by little failures or foibles along the way. You are human after all. Perfection is not a requirement for success.

Find help and support

If you have a supportive family and friends, you are lucky. Being able to talk over your struggles, slip-ups, and goals with those you trust can help immeasurably. Self-help groups can put you in touch with others going through similar experiences. You can learn how others cope and pick up new tricks to help you cope better. Clubs, telephone lines, and health practitioners are all outside sources of help that are available to you.

> *Even without outside support, you can still be successful if quitting smoking is what you want. Your power comes from within you—nowhere else. Only you can change yourself. You must own your life and take responsibility for your destiny, and* **now** *is the right time for you to do it.*

We all make mistakes. Mistakes are nothing more than opportunities to learn something we didn't know before. To use mistakes to your best advantage, try to always make new ones. Try not to make the same mistake twice. And if you do, look at it carefully, learn everything you can from it, and get help if necessary. Trust that you are progressing as you are meant to and that you are guiding your destiny in the direction you want it to go. That is what self-care is all about.

---

1 *See page 127 for more about Change.*

The road to change is a series of successes and missteps. Keeping this in perspective will ultimately deliver you to the destination you seek. When you experience a setback, forgive yourself. Remember, you aren't supposed to be perfect.

> *Once you have made the decision, deep down, that you don't want to be a smoker anymore, the odds are with you for ultimate success. Discover how good life is; how strong you are; how great you feel; how much better you look and smell and everything tastes; and how much money you save after you have successfully, permanently, and forever quit smoking. Do it now!*

Cancer

Cancer. Just say the word and people are terrified. Just thinking or reading about it makes you feel like you are somehow inviting it. It is the second leading cause of death in the United States. Some forms of cancer are preventable, and many forms can be detected early enough to be cured.

> *This disease is caused by a variety of factors, and we are still learning about many of them. Having risk factors does not mean you will get cancer. Conversely, not having risk factors does not mean you won't.*

Lifestyle behaviors cause many cancers. It's those kinds of cancer we are talking about in this book. For example, we know cigarette smoking causes 90 percent of lung cancers and it increases the risk for a number of other cancers, too. Alcoholic intake increases the risk of oral, esophageal, and oropharyngeal cancers. Smoking and alcohol used together increases the risk even more. High-fat diets, and not eating enough fruits, vegetables, and fiber contribute to the development of some cancers. Obesity and lack of exercise seem to contribute to the development of others.

Family history plays a big role because of the passing of genes from one generation to another. Certain cancers seem to run in families. It is believed this is so because codes on the genetic material are passed from generation to generation. These genetic codes "turn on" the production of cancer cells at some point in time. As we more fully understand our genetic code, new treatments to prevent or cure cancer will certainly come. As we learn how to locate these cellular switches and figure out how to turn them off, new treatments and cures will be discovered.

Environmental factors play a role in the development of cancer, too. Unprotected exposure to sunlight (ultraviolet radiation) is associated with skin cancer. Radiation from x-rays may cause cancer if there is too much exposure. Viruses, bacteria, and parasites have been linked to certain cancers. That doesn't mean that if you get these infections, you will get cancer. It just means you may have greater risk if other risks or circumstances are present.

Substances called *carcinogens* increase the risk of getting cancer. We are only beginning to understand the extent to which toxins (or poisons) in our environment are increasing the occurrence of cancers. Substances like pesticides, herbicides, asbestos, arsenic, nickel, nuclear waste, and industrial emissions have all been implicated in causing cancer.

There is just no guarantee when it comes to the development of cancer. It seems to be a random beast. But there are things you can learn about yourself, your family, and your environment to determine if your risk is greater than others. And there are behaviors that will decrease your risks and make you stronger and more able to fight off cancer successfully should it occur.

Are you at risk?

The following questions will show you what you are or are not doing about cancer risk.

Are your cancer screenings such as PAP smear, prostate exam, mammogram, colonoscopy overdue?	❑ Yes	❑ No
Do you need follow-up by a health professional?	❑ Yes	❑ No
Do you smoke?	❑ Yes	❑ No
Do you have a history of any cancers in your family?	❑ Yes	❑ No
Is your Body Mass Index (BMI) greater than 25?	❑ Yes	❑ No
Do you get less than 240 minutes of exercise per week at your target heart rate?	❑ Yes	❑ No

Is your diet high in fat and low in fruits, vegetables, and fiber?	❑ Yes	❑ No
Do you drink more than two alcoholic beverages a day?	❑ Yes	❑ No
Have you had a substantial lifetime sun exposure?	❑ Yes	❑ No

Answering yes to any of these questions demonstrates that you might have risk for cancer.

When reviewing your risk factors, ***remember that having a risk factor does not mean you will get the disease.***

It only means that, when compared with someone without that risk factor, an increased incidence of that cancer has been observed. Some people with multiple risk factors never develop the disease; other people who do develop cancer have no known risk factors for it.

Cancer, in contrast to other conditions discussed in this book, *is not a wholly preventable disease*. Lifestyle behaviors can, and indeed do, strongly influence your risk of certain cancers—we *know* smoking causes lung cancer and contributes to the risk for others. But even the person with the most "perfect" lifestyle behaviors is still at risk for cancer. Your behaviors cannot prevent diseases that are carried in your genes. Your behaviors cannot prevent known or unknown uncontrollable exposures to cancer-causing substances in the workplace or pollutants present in the natural environment. Even those who take great care of themselves are still at risk for cancer.

If diagnosed with cancer, those in good health will do better overall because of their better physical condition. Thus, someone diagnosed with lung cancer in the early stages might have a good chance for complete cure. But if that person is also obese, has heart disease, and chronic lung disease from a lifetime of smoking, the treatment is going to be more dangerous and difficult than if his or her weight, heart, and lungs were in better shape at the time of diagnosis. This is why it is important to be as healthy as possible in your lifestyle choices.

Cancer is a frightening disease in which abnormal cells divide without control. It can occur anywhere in the body and at any age, although 80 percent of cancers occur in people over age 55. Cancer is usually caused by damage to genes that are inside our bodies' cells. Genes are basic parts of our cells that we inherit from our biological parents. They determine our traits—like hair or eye color and risks for certain diseases, including cancers.

Cells affected by cancer are called *malignant*. Malignant cells are different from normal cells. They divide or grow much more rapidly than they should. This rapid division and growth can destroy surrounding body tissues or spread to other parts of the body.

Cancer spreading from an original site to another location in the body is called *metastasis*. When cells divide at an accelerated rate, they sometimes form a mass of tissue called a *tumor*. The tumor is fed by blood vessels that can carry the cancer away to other parts of the body. Tumors can be either malignant or benign.

A malignant tumor is cancerous, and a benign tumor is not. So, not all tumors are cancerous. A benign tumor will not spread (metastasize) to distant parts of the body. Cancer usually forms a tumor, but not always. Leukemia, for example, is cancer in the blood but does not cause tumors.

Understand that different types of cancer behave differently. For example, lung cancer and breast cancer grow at different rates and respond to different treatments. There are more than a hundred different kinds of cancer, and treatments are specific to each particular type of cancer. Some can be screened for, treated early, and cured. The survival rate for these cancers is usually good. Types of treatments, methods of diagnosis, and insurance coverage for testing vary by state and the type of insurance you have. The guidelines below are from the American Cancer Society.

Screening for cancer

Screening tests are done for the purpose of checking for cancer before there are symptoms. Some screenings are self-examinations (like self-breast exams, self-testicular exams, or notifying your healthcare provider of a mole or wart you have noticed changing). Some screenings are part of your physical examination (like a PAP smear and rectal exam). Some screenings are tests that are performed by someone other than your regular health practitioner. For example, a mammogram is done at an x-ray center. A medical specialist called a gastroenterologist performs a colonoscopy.

The American Cancer Society recommends the following cancer

screenings:

- **Breast Cancer.** Self- and clinical-breast exam (performed by your health practitioner) and a yearly mammogram starting at age 40 and continuing as long as a woman is in good health.
- **Cervical Cancer.** Screening PAP smears should begin within three years after a woman begins having vaginal intercourse and no later than age 21. PAPs should be performed every year. After age 30, women who have had three normal PAPs in a row may be screened every two to three years unless they are at high risk (talk to your health professional about your cervical cancer risks). After a total hysterectomy, PAP smears may be discontinued unless cervical cancer was the reason for the hysterectomy. Women over the age of 70 may discontinue PAP smears if they have had three or more normal smears in the prior 10 years.
- **Colon and Rectal Cancer.** A fecal occult blood test every year starting at age 50 and a screening colonoscopy every 5 to 10 years based on the recommendation of the gastroenterologist who performs it.
- **Oral Cancer.** Examination of the mouth by a medical or dental health professional.
- **Prostate Cancer.** Digital rectal exam and PSA (prostate-specific antigen) blood test every year starting at age 50 and continued as long as life expectancy is greater than 10 years. Men at high risk (African Americans and men who have had a relative diagnosed with prostate cancer at a young age) should start screenings at age 45.
- **Skin Cancer.** A skin survey is an examination in which the skin on your entire body is examined under good light and magnification to look for suspicious lesions; biopsies are performed as needed.
- **Testicular Cancer.** Self-testicular exam and a clinical exam performed at routine medical health checkups.

Cancers for which there are screening tests and / or possible preventions

Type of Cancer	Estimated New Cases Per Year	Estimated Deaths Per Year
Skin Cancer – all	1,300,000	10,000
(Melanoma only)	(59,940)	(8,110)

Lung Cancer (2nd for men *and* women combined)	213,380	160,390
Breast Cancer	180,510	40,910
Prostate Cancer	218,890	27,050
Colorectal Cancer	153,760	52,870
Head and Neck Cancer	34,360	7,550
Cervical Cancer	11,150	3,670
Testicular Cancer	7,920	380

American Cancer Society: Cancer Facts and Figures, 2007

For certain types of cancers, there is no screening to detect them until they begin to cause symptoms. And one of the most frightening aspects of certain cancers is that they may not cause any symptoms until late in the disease process.

Cancers for which there are no current screening tests

Type of Cancer	Estimated New Cases Per Year	Estimated Deaths Per Year
Lymphoma	71,380	19,730
Bladder Cancer	67,160	13,750
Kidney Cancer	51,190	12,890
Leukemia (all types)	44,240	21,790
Uterine Cancer	39,080	7,400
Pancreatic Cancer	37,170	33,370
Thyroid Cancer	33,550	1,530
Ovarian Cancer	22,430	15,280
Stomach Cancer	21,260	11,210
Brain Cancer	20,500	12,740
Multiple Myeloma	19,900	10,790
Liver Cancer	19,160	16,780

American Cancer Society: Cancer Facts and Figures, 2007

Cancer is a bit like a wild beast. You never really know when it will lie down or when it will strike. The best way to protect yourself is to work with your healthcare provider to get regular screening and take good care of yourself. A little prayer won't hurt either.

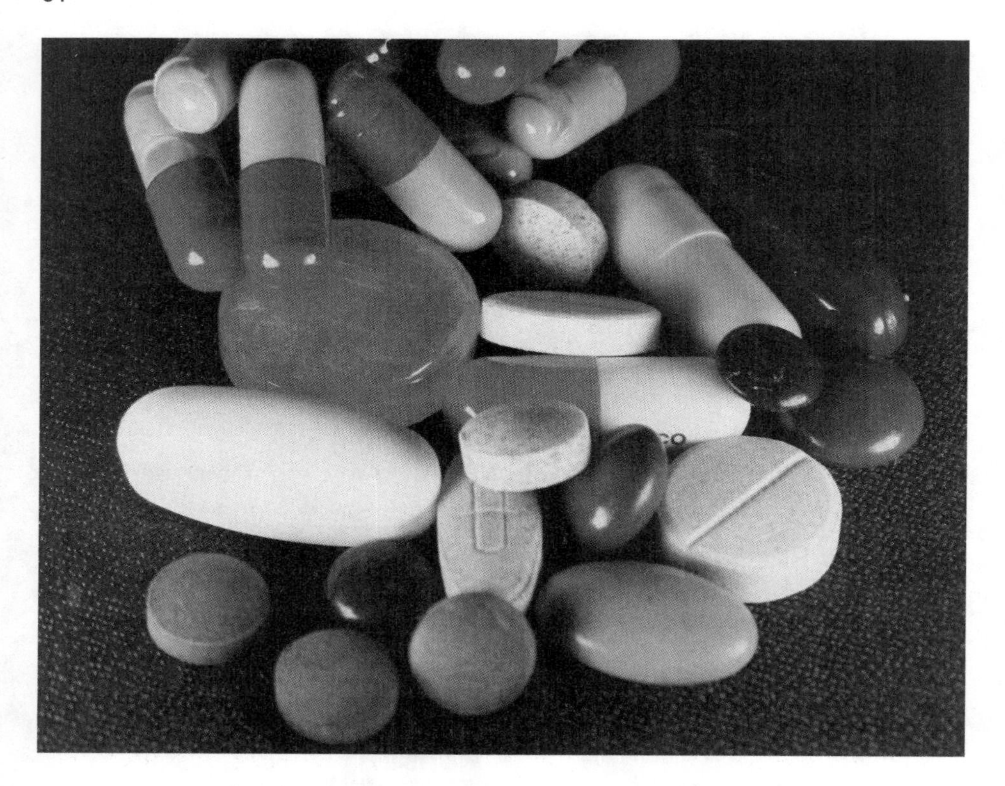

Medications and Your Health

Many of the conditions discussed so far in this book require both medications *and* lifestyle change. And while there is a common perception that taking meds is a sign of being unhealthy—that is incorrect. Uncontrolled health risks are what are unhealthy—not the medications that treat and control them. If your health practitioner recommends medication, you should listen and be open minded about the possible benefits. Yes, taking pills every day may seem like a heavy burden. But, which burden is heavier, taking pills every day or suffering from illness?

You should neither ignore the need for medication, nor turn to medication to cure every ill. It is your responsibility to learn everything you can about medications that are recommended or prescribed for you and any you purchase over the counter. Medications are tools. Used properly they are life-prolonging and life-saving.

The benefit of medication for chronic and acute health problems is undisputed. Yet nowhere is there more frustration and miscommunication between health practitioners and their patients than where medications are concerned. And nowhere is there a greater need for a trusting relationship and clear understanding between you and your prescribing practitioner than where medications are concerned.

Many patients want medications from their health practitioners (like antibiotics) when they are not recommended and will not be effective. At the same time, many resist medications that are recommended for chronic conditions like high blood pressure or high cholesterol, believing (incorrectly) that it's bad to have to take medications regularly. The fact is most health risks come from the untreated conditions—not the medications that treat them.

If you find that you do need to be on a medication regimen, it is imperative—***imperative***—that you learn to take your medications exactly as prescribed. Even if you are simply taking an over-the-counter drug, this same principle applies. Medications are carefully dosed. This dosage is determined by a professional. You are not that professional. Do not assume that when it comes to medication you know more than that professional.

There are thousands of different medications, and they work in many different ways in the body. Understanding some of the different ways medications work will help you alleviate the fear of being medication dependant. This same understanding can also help you to become a wiser medication user. The following are some of the common ways medications work. They illustrate how your compliance with a dosing schedule affects how effective the medication will be. This is by no means a comprehensive review of all the different ways drugs work in the body, but it should serve to clarify some of the biggest misunderstandings about commonly used drugs and how they need to be taken.

Antibiotics are drugs that kill bacteria that cause infections. There are two kinds of germs that cause infection: bacteria and viruses. Antibiotics *only* kill bacteria; they are not effective against viruses. The common cold and the flu (influenza) are viruses. There is no antibiotic that cures a cold or the flu. Antibiotics cure bacterial infections by killing specific bacterial organisms that cause the illness. Antibiotics work by being in the bloodstream long enough and at high enough concentrations to kill all the bacteria. The dose your health practitioner prescribes is not random. It has been determined by how much (what dose), how long (number of days of treatment), and how often (number of doses a day) it takes to kill all the bacteria causing your infection. If it's the wrong drug, it won't kill the germs. If it's the wrong dose, it won't kill the germs. If it isn't taken long enough, it won't kill all the germs. Every time you are prescribed antibiotics, you should take every single pill (as many times a day as ordered) and then throw away the empty bottle. You should never have antibiotics left over. You should never share antibiotics, because then neither of you will have enough medication to cure the infection.

"As needed" medications like Tylenol (acetaminophen), Advil / Motrin (ibuprofen), Aleve (naprosyn), pain medications, cold medications, and others are taken only when needed. If you have a headache or cold, or bang your thumb with a hammer, you take this type of medication. When your discomfort or symptoms resolve, you stop taking it.

Steady-state medications are drugs that are only effective at certain blood levels. These drugs require occasional blood tests to check their levels in the bloodstream. If there is not enough of the drug in the bloodstream, the drug will not have the desired effect. Conversely, if there is too much of the drug in the bloodstream, it can have dangerous side effects. Examples of drugs of this type include digoxin for the heart, Dilantin for seizures, Coumadin for blood thinning, and theophylline for lung disease.

> *To maintain steady levels of drugs in the bloodstream, they must be taken without fail and with absolute regularity.*

Usually a loading dose is required when the drug is first started to get the blood levels up to where the drug can have its effect. This loading dose is larger than the usual daily dose. Every time a dose of this type of drug is missed, the blood level drops a little. This greatly affects whether the drug works in the system. People who take these drugs diligently only need their blood tested occasionally to check their levels. Those who do not take their medications properly have to have blood tests more often to keep their levels where they should be so the drug can be effective.

Maintenance medications are what you take regularly to treat or prevent chronic conditions. These medications are usually required for extended periods, and often for life.

They can prevent illness and its complications, but must be taken exactly as ordered and with unwavering faithfulness if they are to do you the most good. Blood pressure, cholesterol, diabetic, psychiatric, asthma, heart, and lung medications all fall into this category.

Sometimes people resist these types of medications, mistakenly believing they are somehow "healthier" without them. This is wrong. If a medication has been appropriately prescribed, it will extend your life and improve your health. If you stop taking the drug after it has done its job, the health problem the drug was controlling will return.

If you are opposed to a medication for any reason, you should be very honest and open with your practitioner about your feelings.

It is always *your* decision whether or not to take a medication. It is a mistake to leave your practitioner in the dark about your intentions. Speak up if you don't like, can't afford, don't believe in, or have side effects from any medication that is recommended. Medications are offered to benefit you. If you feel they offer you none, say so. You need to be very clear on why you believe the prescribed meds aren't for you. And you need to listen carefully to your health practitioner's reasons for offering them. Only then can you make an informed decision that is right for you.

If you do accept the responsibility of a medication regimen, remember, it is just that—*a responsibility*. You accept the task of making certain your medication is taken correctly all of the time. You are also responsible for making sure that you don't run out of medication and knowing what you can and can't take, eat, or drink with that medication. Accidents happen. But the best way to protect yourself is to *know your medications.*

Be informed about your medications

You should know the following about every medication you take, including nonprescription medications:

- **Both the brand and generic names of the medication.** (The brand name is capitalized, the generic name is not.)
- **What it looks like.** You should be able to identify all the medications you take. If you do not recognize a pill you are given, question it *before* you take it.
- **Why you take it.** ("Because my doctor told me to" is *not* why.)
- **The dose you are on and how often you should take it.**
- **The time of day you should take it.**
- **Any side effects you should watch for** and what to do if you have them.
- **Any interactions with other medications you take or with foods.**
- **Any special instructions.** For example, other medications to avoid, whether to take with food or on an empty stomach, whether to avoid sun exposure, etc.
- **If any new medication duplicates anything you are already taking.**

Don't make the mistake of not taking the time to learn everything you can about your medications. You should keep a complete list of all the medications you are currently taking (including doses) with you at all times. The days when you could leave things up to your health professionals are over. Likely more than one health practitioner will treat you over time, and you must be able to give each one a complete medication list.

> *Having a list of all your medications will help your health providers give you better care and will reduce your risk of suffering a medication error.*

One type of medication error you should be aware of is called *poly-pharmacy*. This is a case of being on too many medications that are working at cross-purposes to each other. When you are seen by multiple health professionals, as is common in today's world of specialization, you will have multiple practitioners prescribing medications for you. If you don't know what you are taking, how can you inform them?

To prevent poly-pharmacy keep a current and complete medication list with you at all times. This is the most beneficial thing you can do for your health and healthcare. It will help practitioners see how others are treating you. Then you can both make the best decision for you. If you have questions, it is a good idea to put all your medicine and vitamin bottles in a bag and take them with you to your appointment. Medication labels have a lot of useful information that will help your health provider when reviewing your medications.

There is no reason to be afraid of treatment with a number of medications so long as they are appropriately prescribed. Certain conditions, like high blood pressure, may require three or even four medications to reach target numbers. Likewise, heart disease, diabetes, and certain psychiatric conditions may require combinations of medications to reach goals and achieve therapeutic results. Staying informed about all your medications and keeping an up-to-date medication list becomes even more important here.

Managing medications is one of the reasons why everyone should have a primary care practitioner who oversees all the healthcare you receive. This person will keep an eye on the big picture. Sometimes, medications can be combined or eliminated. Sometimes, you may be on more than one of the same type of medicine. If two different health practitioners have prescribed and didn't have the benefit of your complete medication list when they treated you, there is a greater risk of this.

Do not stop medications without consulting your practitioner. Some medications should be tapered off slowly, and others should not be stopped at all. Don't take risks with your health or your medications. Partnership with your practitioner and good communication will help you get the most benefit from your medications and reduce the risks of poly-pharmacy and other med errors.

Medications are valuable tools developed over long periods of time and have undergone years of testing and study. For the most part, they are safe when taken correctly under the supervision of a health professional.

Now that you have the information you need to assess your health risks, it's time to talk about choice and changes you can make to improve your health.

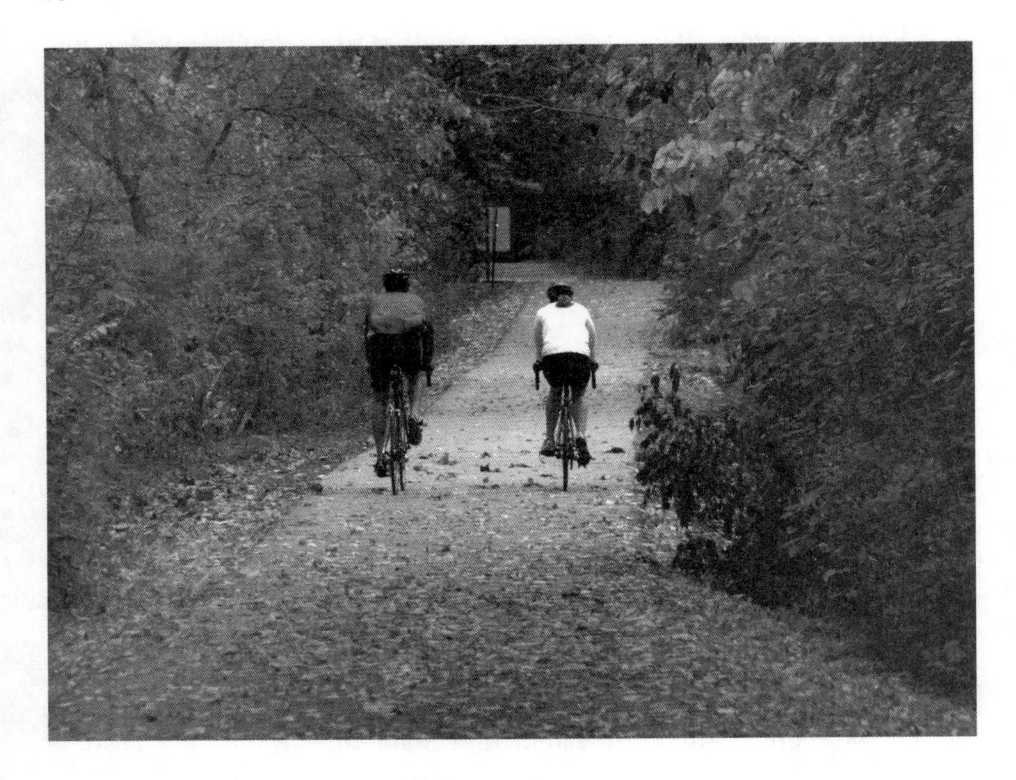

Your First Choice: *Exercise*

Have you seen a repeating theme through this book so far? Have you noticed that all of the lifestyle changes that will reduce risk started first and foremost with the addition of an exercise program? Don't moan, you've known this to be true for many years. Admit it.

The advice to exercise is not new and shocking. We have known for hundreds and hundreds of years that physical vitality is critically linked to health. The human body is designed for movement, and it declines quickly if it is not constantly challenged.

Exercise will promote your health and happiness more than any other single activity.

There is no part of your health and life that will not be improved by a regimen of regular physical activity. The improvements you will enjoy as a result of exercise are hard to imagine if you have not been physically active.

Movement is Life

Watch schoolchildren on the playground. They don't go out to run, yet they can't help spontaneously breaking into a run. They sprint here, and they sprint there. They run, they stop, they chase things and each other, and they throw and catch things. They are in constant motion. Their movement is unstructured and unplanned; it is completely natural.

Once we go to school and work, most of us become physically imprisoned. Whether sitting at our desks or in cars or airplanes, or being stationary at some task for hours, our bodies are not moving, stretching, and strengthening. Even jobs that were once physically intensive are now automated. Machines and tools do much of the work that was once done with the body.

As we grow up, we gradually lose the spontaneous movement of childhood. The less we move, the less we want to move. Left idle, our bodies become more and more immobile. As our bodies gradually become less fluid and flexible, pains and body aches develop. Our weight begins to increase because we do nothing to burn up the food we take in. That makes us even less inclined to move around. This is how the cycle of immobility and uncontrollable weight gain begins. For many, the cycle is never broken, and the body literally runs down from lack of use.

Exercise can be found in the simplest of places. Yes, you should begin an exercise program that is above and beyond what you do already during the day. But you can easily add some physical activity to your day with just the barest of adjustments.

Don't look for the closest parking spot. Park far away and walk to the stores. Or take the stairs instead of the elevator. Take a bike to work if you can. Walk somewhere instead of driving. These are just a few, minor adjustments that can help you get into a habit of exercise. Alone, they are certainly not enough to make the difference you need to turn a risk into a chance. But they will get the ball rolling. And that just might be all it takes.

According to the National Center for Health Statistics, only one-third of adults report that they are participating in regular and sustained physical activity during their leisure time. Those who are exercising have already discovered how much life improves with regular activity.

How much exercise is enough?

The **American College of Sports Medicine (ACSM)** and the **American Heart Association (AHA)** guidelines were last updated in August 2007 and recommend that all healthy adults engage in regular aerobic endurance exercise.

The minimum amount of time recommended is 30 minutes, 5 days a week for activities performed at the lower end of your target heart rate. For more vigorous activities performed at the higher end of your target heart rate, the minimum amount of time recommended is 20 minutes, 3 days a week. In addition, strength training should be performed a minimum of two days per week. The guidelines state that for improved fitness, to reduce your risk of chronic disease and prevent weight gain—more is better! This book recommends a ***minimum*** *of 240 minutes of exercise per week performed at your target heart rate.*

How Hard Should You Exercise?

The level of *intensity* for a physical activity is measured by the *percent of your maximum heart rate* required to perform it. You can estimate your maximum heart rate by subtracting your age from 220. To find the heart rate you want to sustain during exercise, you multiply your maximum heart rate times 60 percent and 80 percent to get your target heart rate range during exercise. Use the following example (but insert your current age):

- If, for example, you are 50 years old, then:

  220 – 50 = 170 beats per minute = your maximum heart rate

- If you reach a heart rate during exercise of 170 beats per minute, you are exercising at 100 percent of your maximum heart rate. You would be unable to sustain this level of exertion for long.

  170 X 60% (.60) = 102 beats per minute

  102 beats per minute is the minimum target heart rate for when you are exercising. If your heart rate isn't at least 102, you are not getting aerobic or conditioning benefit from your exercise.

  170 X 80% (.80) = 136 beats per minute

136 beats per minute is the upper limit of the target heart rate for when you are exercising. As you become more fit, you will become more comfortable exercising at this higher percentage of your maximum heart rate.

At 50 years old, you want to exercise most days of the week for between 30 and 60 minutes keeping your heart rate between 102 and 136 beats per minute the whole time.

How do you count your heart rate?

You count your heart rate by feeling your pulse. There are two easy places on your body to do this, and you can do either at rest or while you are exercising.

You can feel for your pulse on one side of your neck next to your Adam's apple (don't feel both sides of your Adam's apple at the same time, as that can trigger irregular heartbeats). The other easy place to feel a pulse is on your wrist just below the palm at the base of your thumb. Press two or three fingers down until you feel the pulse, and then lighten your touch until you can easily feel the pulse beating and can count the beats.

Count the pulse for 6 seconds and multiply the number by 10 (6 seconds x 10 = 60 seconds = 1 minute). For example, if you feel 12 beats of your pulse in 6 seconds and multiply that number times 10, it equals 120 beats per minute. That means (if you are 50 years old) you are in your target heart rate range between 102 and 136 (working at 60 percent to 80 percent of your maximum heart rate). If you can maintain that heart rate for 30 to 60 minutes, you are getting the recommended exercise for your heart for that exercise session.

To elevate your heart rate, you must move large muscles of your body like your arms and legs; this way you are also exercising and conditioning your muscles at the same time you are conditioning your heart. As a result, your respirations will become more rapid in order to increase the amount of oxygen flowing to your heart and muscles. This conditions your body to use oxygen more efficiently. As you continue to exercise and as you become more fit, all these processes will become easier and more efficient, and will not require the same level of exertion that you feel when you first start out.

How Do You Get Started?

See your health practitioner: Men over age 40 and women over age 50 (women's health risks increase after they go through menopause), all smokers, and those with chronic illnesses who plan to begin a new program of vigorous activity should have a physical examination before beginning an exercise program.

During your appointment, you will want to review your health risks and medical history. This is particularly important if you have chronic health problems such as heart disease, high blood pressure or diabetes, or if you find through reading this book that you are at high risk for any of these conditions.

The purpose of a medical evaluation prior to starting an exercise program is to uncover any health conditions that might be made worse by exercise. Because the purpose of exercise includes stressing and strengthening the heart, a key part of a medical evaluation will focus on the health of the heart.

Other medical considerations are:

- Muscular or skeletal problems such as arthritis or injuries that may play a role in choosing which activities are best for you.
- Certain illnesses like hepatitis may make contact sports inadvisable so as to prevent inadvertent blows to the liver or spleen.
- Skin infections might need to be treated prior to participating in contact sports like wrestling.
- Conditions such as poor circulation or asthma may limit a person's exercise tolerance or require medications to help with athletic performance.

Remember, exercise is a health-promoting, not dangerous, activity if approached with common sense.

Those people who suffer adverse medical events from exercise are extremely rare. If you have not been active, you should start with short sessions (5–10 minutes) of physical activity and gradually build up to your desired level of fitness. Any new physical activity should be built up slowly to prevent muscle strains or injuries. A little soreness goes along with any new physical activity; outright pain is something else and should be evaluated by a medical professional. And don't expect yourself to become a warrior athlete overnight.

Symptoms that require immediate attention

*The following are symptoms you should **not** ignore and for which you should **seek immediate medical attention:***

- **Chest pain or pressure,** an ache in the jaw or neck, discomfort down the left or right arms, pain across the shoulders and back.
- **Unaccustomed or unusual shortness of breath** (If you have been inactive and begin to exercise for the first time, shortness of breath is normal. If it seems abnormal to you, seek medical attention.)
- **Dizziness or lightheadedness.**
- **Heart rhythm abnormalities.**

The Best Regimen

Find your primary exercise activity. This is what you will put time into faithfully—through good times and bad, good weather and bad, whether you're in the mood or not. This is the activity you are going to "Just Do." Choose walking, running, biking, swimming, or some combination.

Put in at least 240 minutes a week, faithfully. Get your heart rate up to its target level based on your age. At the beginning, you may have to work through some mental and physical resistance. In time it will get easier, and, eventually, your exercise sessions could turn out to be the very best part of your day.

Aim for 20 to 30 minutes of yoga or some form of stretching most days. After every aerobic workout is an ideal time because your muscles are warm and will appreciate the stretch. If you have no knowledge of yoga, join a class until you understand how to do it and can practice on your own with good form.

Finally, if you are walking, running, biking, or swimming, get to a gym and check out some free weights. Learn how to lift weights with good form. Concentrate on your upper body. Your legs will likely be strengthened with the exercise of your aerobic activity. Once you know how to lift with good form, purchase some free weights to use at home. I recommend 15-, 12-, 10-, 8-, 5-, and 3-pound weights for women. Men will need heavier weights. Aim for three weight sessions per week.

Join the gym if you will enjoy it and work out three days a week. Find an instructional book or program (I like Bill Phillip's *Body for Life*) to inspire you.

If you can afford it, a private trainer for three to six months (or forever) will teach you a lot about exercise. The one-on-one attention and the change you will see and feel in your body over those months may get you hooked on exercise for life. And that's the goal!

If you like company, find a friend who will exercise with you.

To embrace physical activity in your life does not mean you must hang out in a gym pushing heavy weights, run a marathon, or put on spandex and go to an aerobics class (though there are those who will find some of those activities appealing). You can exercise vigorously at home, or on the road, with little or no equipment. The secret is to get yourself turned on!

Be inspired by female body builders who went to gyms for the very first time as frail elderly ladies trying to fight osteoporosis. They got turned on to weight lifting and started participating in weight-lifting competitions in their 70s!

Or how about the non-athletes who never played a sport in their lives, and took up jogging because it is easy and they wanted to lose weight? They got turned on; they trained and began competing in marathons.

There are others who went to their first aerobics class, got turned on, and went on to become aerobics instructors themselves.

Are you a sports fan? Do you like baseball? Join a softball league and field some grounders yourself. You'll appreciate the pros even more.

Follow tennis? Go play yourself. It makes watching the pros a lot more fun, and you'll learn from them how to improve your own game.

Watch golf? If you play, too, have you trained your body to play your best and strongest round?

> *Life is not a spectator sport. Be the superstar of your own life. Leave yourself open to getting turned on to something—anything—active.*

Remember, the secret to a happy life is *balance.* You need activity and you need rest. Rest allows the body to recover from activity. With every period of exertion there is a breakdown of bodily tissues, and with every period of rest there is repair of the body to a stronger state than it was before the exertion. There must be enough exercise for the body to strengthen. There must be enough rest for the body to repair. You will find your own proper balance. Exercise enough to get steadily stronger and healthier, while allowing enough time to rest and keep you energized and eager to continue.

> *Exercise is fertilizer for the body. Use it to grow strong, vigorous, and energetic.*

Motivation is the primary and essential ingredient you will need to get yourself moving. Motivation is what drives and steers change. If you are not motivated, you will not succeed no matter what your goal. Find your motivation before attempting any change including starting an exercise program. It is the rocket fuel that will power your ascent. This book has been written to motivate you, educate you, and empower you. If you are not moved to action right now, why not? Can you picture yourself the way you want to be? Then you are ready and able to change. Take your vision and allow it to be your guiding light. It can become your precious motivation.

Past experience is a tremendous motivator. If you have ever made a change in the past, you can use what you learned about yourself then to make any new change successful now. Everything you experience and everything you learn in life increases your skill level. The more skills you have, the better your chances of success. So keep learning, keep experiencing. Even if you cannot manage this change, you'll enjoy a richer life.

Time will support you in the process of change. The best way to use it is to set aside a specific period of time during which you are willing to commit 100 percent to your goal. You need to stick with it for at least 12 weeks before you can determine success. Commit for 12 weeks and see where they take you.

Show up every day. Take small victories; don't focus on winning the whole war. Change should happen in small, permanent steps that add up to success over time. Remember, you are growing a habit of daily exercise. One day you will turn around and your whole world will be changed, and you'll wonder when it finally happened. So think your of goals like stepping stones. Keep putting small steps in front of you and keep taking them. Later you can look back at the lovely path you have created.

Be prepared. To stay on track as you work toward this goal, arrange your environment so that it offers support and does not remind you of your old habits or behaviors. Let that reinforce what it is you want to change. If you want to exercise in the morning before work, lay your exercise clothes out before you go to bed so that they are waiting for you in the morning. Don't stay up too late so that when the alarm goes off you are rested and ready for your workout.

Find things that support your effort, like a personal trainer, or a good friend with whom you can exercise or eat better meals. Half the task, half the effort.

> *Reward yourself with something that reinforces your changed behavior. Buy new sneakers or a workout outfit. You should feel rewarded all along the way. Enjoying an activity that opposes the behavior you are trying to banish should fill you with great joy and accomplishment.*

Remember, exercise is a choice and a change for the better. It will rescue you from many ills. Make exercise your friend. It will serve you all your days.

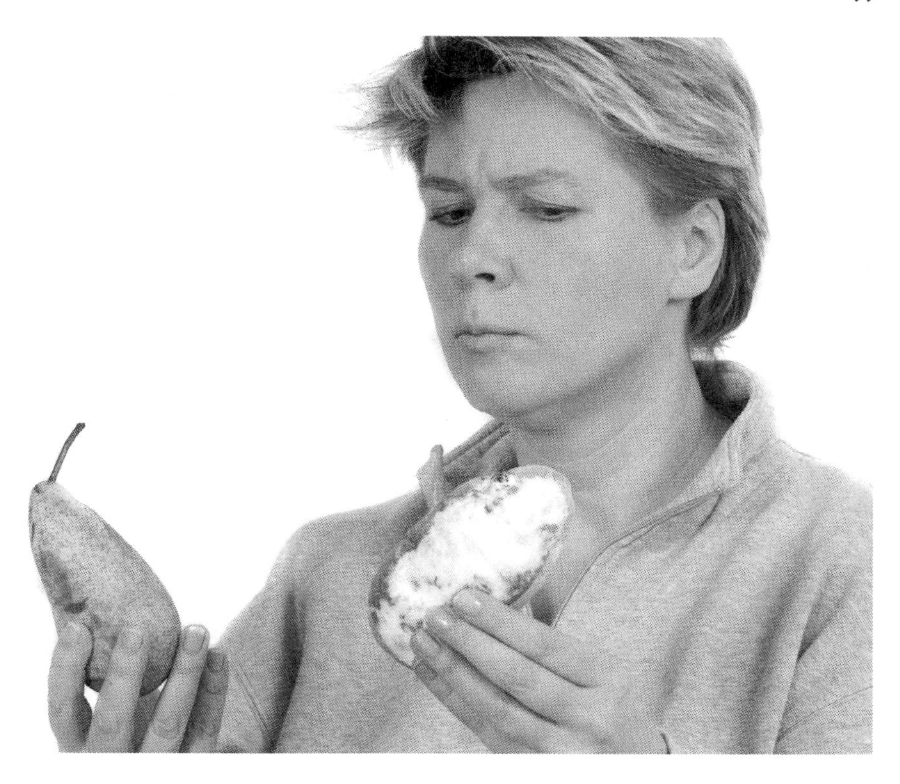

Your Second Choice: *Weight and Nutrition*

There is a common thread that runs through the fabric of chronic disease. That is, it may be preventable, and it is certainly controllable, and both are accomplished with your behaviors. The need for exercise and the need to maintain a healthy body weight are both essential. These two healthy behaviors will do more for your health and quality of life than you can possibly imagine. You've heard it before. You'll hear it again. That's because it's true. If you want to be healthy, you must exercise. And you must control your weight. Sorry. But that's that. There are no other long-term solutions.

> *Excess body weight is not merely a cosmetic problem. It is a health risk, and it contributes to every other health risk in this book.*

People who are overweight are twice as likely to die prematurely as those whose weights are normal. Being overweight causes one-half of all the cases of high blood pressure and triples the risk of developing diabetes. A study published in the *New England Journal of Medicine* found that 1 in every 6 cancer deaths could be prevented by losing weight. Three hundred thousand deaths every year are in some way associated with being overweight.

Nearly two-thirds of the adults in the United States are overweight—that's about 97 million people. Nearly 25 percent of American adults are obese, meaning they have a Body Mass Index greater than 30. About 15 percent of children and adolescents are now overweight. Of those, about 70 percent will remain overweight and obese as adults. Obesity is increasing in every state in the United States; in men, women, and children; across all races, all age groups, all educational levels. We are all gaining weight so uncontrollably that the Surgeon General predicts excess weight will overtake smoking as the number one cause of preventable death within the next 10 years.

The subject of weight is a sensitive one. Our media-driven body ideals make it so difficult for people to be comfortable in the bodies they have. It generates stress and a defeatist attitude about the realities of weight and weight management. Oftentimes, people give up entirely, believing that they will never make the ideal and, therefore, are absolved of the effort completely. Or they go to extremes and starve the body of what it vitally needs. In these instances, weight is not a health issue; it is a vanity one.

Overweight does not mean just carrying a few extra pounds. As a matter of fact, let's forget about pounds completely. That is an image-driven conception. We need to shift our understanding of weight away from simple image perception and into a genuine health concern. Being overweight means more than being unable to buy fashionable clothes. Being overweight means that your body is under strain from simply carrying itself around.

Excess weight serves no physiologic purpose. It puts a strain on all the systems of the body. Think of taking a quantity of bricks equal to the number of pounds you are overweight and putting them in a bag. Imagine having to carry that bag of bricks everywhere you go and never being able to put it down. Carrying a 10- or 15-pound bag everywhere you go would become exhausting even before the end of a single day.

The strain of excess weight affects all the systems of the body. The heart has to work harder. The lungs have to work harder. (Think of how you huff and puff when you have to carry a heavy load up a flight of stairs.) The bones and muscles have to hold up and support the extra weight. Because of excess fat in the body, cholesterol and other fats tend to build up in the bloodstream and around organs. Certain cells, like those with insulin receptors, become insensitive because of the excess fat; blood sugar rises, and diabetes can result. Excess body fat can increase the risks of certain cancers, believe it or not.

To get a feeling for the overall strain on your system, try this experiment. Take a weight that feels heavy to you and lift it 8 to 10 times. At the end of the reps you may have had to struggle to continue lifting it. Now, put that weight down and pick up another weight that feels light. Lift it 8 or 10 times. Feel how much easier that is? That is how much easier your whole body can function once you lose the excess weight. Everything gets easier.

Are you at risk?

If you answer yes to one or more of the following statements, you are at risk from your weight. Recognizing it is not shameful. This is a boat that many, many people are rowing together. The question becomes then, are you going to make the second choice, or let it ride right by? Be honest with yourself here, and know that this is a problem that can be solved.

I am female and my waist measurement is greater than 35 inches. I am male and my waist measurement is greater than 40 inches.	❏ Yes	❏ No
My diet is high fat with lots of fast or fried foods and / or baked goods.	❏ Yes	❏ No

I can control my weight only by constant effort and struggle.	❑ Yes	❑ No
My eating is out of control.	❑ Yes	❑ No
My eating patterns and relationship to food are very uncomfortable.	❑ Yes	❑ No
My daily activities are limited by my weight.	❑ Yes	❑ No
As a child I was overweight or obese.	❑ Yes	❑ No
One or both of my parents were (or are) overweight or obese.	❑ Yes	❑ No

Knowing is half the battle. But, if pounds are no indication of a healthy weight, and a visual determination of obesity is irrelevant, then how do we know if our weight is healthy?

The standard of measure for obesity is called the *Body Mass Index*. Body mass index (BMI) measures body fat based on both weight and height. See page 210 to determine your BMI. Scientific study has shown that your health risks increase when your BMI is greater than 25. For that reason, we will use a BMI of less than or equal to 25 as our goal for reducing health risks from excess weight.

However, not everyone is the same size. There are many people for whom a target BMI of 25 is not realistic. If a BMI of less than 25 is not reasonable for you, it does not mean you should abandon efforts if weight loss is needed. The loss of 10 percent to 15 percent of your total body weight will pay huge health benefits and can dramatically improve your life and reduce your health risks.

Losing weight is not easy. It is a long-term process that takes patience and time. There really is no quick fix. Your genes play a large role in how you wear your weight, and they will also determine how quickly you lose that weight. You might lose weight and still be a large person. That does not mean that you should accept defeat, believing that you will never be healthy and fit. Weight is only one aspect of a healthy body, and there is no one magic method for everybody. There is no standard of perfect body weight.

An all-or-nothing attitude will not help you where excess weight is concerned. If you think you can't be healthy until you lose 50 pounds, you are wrong. Fitness is what counts. If you undertake the effort to lose whatever weight you can and add cardiovascular exercise, you are already on the road to risk reduction.

> *Being heavy and fit is actually healthier than being skinny and unfit! Don't be ashamed of your size. Treat yourself to the same self-care you would if you were the embodiment of your idea of perfection. That will get you closest to becoming the perfect you.*

You may simply not have the genetic makeup to be skinny. And our cultural ideal of emaciated thinness is not a healthy or realistic one, so abandon that idea gratefully. You want to be healthy and fit! You want to be the right size for you. You want to find a diet that allows your body to come back into balance with itself. Proper nutrition in the proper amount will bring you back to center.

If you can get to a BMI of 25 through healthy diet and exercise, go for it. If that is not a realistic target for you, aim for fitness. Even if you are heavy, your pursuit of fitness will lower your blood pressure and cholesterol, prevent diabetes, and protect you from cardiovascular disease. In addition, you will enjoy the pleasures of movement, which is something many people who are heavy miss out on.

There is a simple truth about weight gain and weight loss that will never change.

> *The difference between calories consumed and calories expended determines weight gain or weight loss in the human body.*

Shift that balance and you will lose or gain weight according to your behavior. You don't need a fad diet, special foods, or private chef. All you have to do is alter your behavior according to the above ratio to achieve your desired result of weight gain or weight loss. We have already talked about the benefits of movement and exercise. Compound just some simple activity with a shift in how you eat, and weight loss will happen.

If you can set all the fad-diet, quick-loss hype aside, this solution to weight control is actually very simple. The execution of that simple solution can be challenging, though, if you are looking for quick fixes instead of a healthy way to live. The fact is, with a few simple changes to what you are doing right now, you can lose all the weight you want if you are willing to give it time. You do not have to run marathons or do 100 pushups. Something as simple as switching to one percent milk or using low-fat or fat-free condiments like mustard and fat-free mayonnaise can result in weight loss.

If you eat less than you burn up, you will lose weight. If you eat more than you burn up, you will gain weight. If you eat the same amount that you burn up, your weight will not change. To lose weight, you must eat less (take in less energy) and exercise more (burn up more energy). It's that simple.

There are no magic shortcuts. It is not easy to lose weight. At the end of the day it is calorie restriction and increased activity—nothing else takes the weight off. You don't need special foods—you can eat anything you want—as long as you don't eat too many calories.

Long-term weight loss depends on your readiness to adopt lifestyle changes to achieve your goals.

Mental preparation is key, and having reasonable expectations will increase your chances of success. Modest weight loss—equivalent to 10 percent of your body weight—is a good place to start for most people whose BMI lies between 26 and 30. If you keep the weight off, even this modest weight loss will result in fewer years that you might suffer hypertension, diabetes, and / or high cholesterol. It will also reduce your risk of heart attack and stroke. For many people, losing weight will ease the pain of arthritis and improve mobility overall.

But the weight loss we most need will come slowly. You want to burn fat, not muscle. Some of the most popular diets are not healthy. They may show you a significant drop in pounds, but where did those pounds come from? Depriving your body of certain healthful foods can cause it to turn against itself, actually digesting its own protein. Good, healthy weight loss comes from a diet that is balanced and nutritious. By staying true to this philosophy, the weight loss will be easier, and last longer.

The healthiest diet is one that:

- Is high in fruits and vegetables.
- Is low in fat and calories.
- Has adequate protein for tissue growth and repair.

- Is low in sugar and sodium.
- Has plenty of fiber to keep you feeling full and not hungry, to help lower your cholesterol, and to keep your bowels functioning regularly.
- Has plenty of water—not soft drinks, coffee, or alcohol—simple water to replace what we lose and to cleanse our bodies of wastes and other harmful substances.

The variety of healthy, nourishing food available to us every day is a banquet at which we should feast with pleasure, not guilt. Fad diets are characterized by eliminating some food group or type of food with the claim that an evil food group (rather than the total calories taken in) is responsible for weight gain. They promise that you can eat endlessly from the foods on their diet, so long as you banish foods from the "evil" food group. You often find that this food group is something you might need, and the complete banishment of it makes the diet so hard to maintain that you simply abandon it. The reason most fad diets ultimately fail is because they are restrictive in ways that are unnatural. The body rebels and you give up.

In spite of the overwhelming weight problem in our country, sensible advice on diet and nutrition is hard to hear over the roar of fad diets and promises of quick weight loss that are always being sold to us. Many of us are so stressed by food—either the abundance of it or self-imposed restrictions from it—that we can't establish a comfortable relationship with it. Our focus is not on healthy weight management, but quick and easy weight loss. Creating the belief that you can lose weight with no effort is asking to fail.

The following is a list of the popular diets currently in circulation. Some are realistic and effective. Others are just a flash of fat in the fire.

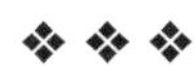

High-Protein / Low-Carbohydrate Diets

Atkins, The Zone, Protein Power

With this diet type you can eat all the meat and fat you want. You can have bacon, sausage, marbled meats, and butter, but you must not eat carbohydrates. So breads, cereals, potatoes, rice, and pastas are all forbidden on this diet. You can have hamburgers, but no bun. You can have bacon and eggs, but no toast.

These diets result in quicker than normal weight loss. The catch is that it is *mostly water and muscle mass that you lose, not fat*. That's because these diets put you into a state of *ketosis*. That means the body is burning up muscle tissue instead of carbohydrates for energy. And ketosis is very rough on the kidneys. These diets also encourage eating high-fat and high-cholesterol meals. This can be dangerous for people with already high cholesterol levels and increases the risk of heart disease and stroke. The diets are deficient in carbohydrates (including fruits and vegetables that are known to lower the risk of cardiovascular disease and some cancers), fiber, and essential vitamins.

Most people don't stick with this kind of diet. Its lack of variety and banishment of so many nutritious and satisfying foods is difficult to sustain permanently. Most people go off it after awhile and then rapidly gain back whatever weight they lost—sometimes even more. This sets up the yo-yo dieting cycle that is so demoralizing and unhealthy.

The appeal of the low-carb craze is that supposedly you can lose weight while eating as much as you want of the high-fat foods that are usually limited in a more balanced weight loss plan. The truth is, the only reason you lose weight with low-carb diets is the same reason you lose on any diet: you take in fewer calories. Ask yourself, when was the last time you got something for nothing?

Low-carb versions of carbohydrates are foods that are produced by a process that leeches out the natural carbs (along with their nutrients) and replaces them with chemicals. You are then charged two to three times the amount you'd pay for the simple whole food all for the privilege of eating the chemicals. Save your money.

The truth is carbohydrates are good for you. Aside from refined sugars and flours where all the nutrients are removed and nothing but the empty calories remain, carbs should not be demonized. Save your money and use your common sense. Banishing carbohydrates from your diet will not make you thin. Sensible eating from all food groups, watching your portion sizes and total calories, plus getting regular exercise is what will allow you to control your weight and eat comfortably and enjoyably. Low-carb diets do have some benefits for certain individuals. For example, they are very useful to diabetics as they do a very good job of controlling blood sugars. They help stabilize insulin secretion and blood sugar swings. This is largely because a low-carb diet will take you off refined flour and sweets like baked goods, which are high in refined sugar. However, if you just limit white flour, baked sweets, and sugar in your diet, you will achieve the same effect without eliminating a whole healthy food group.

Very Low Fat Diet: Dean Ornish

This is a diet prescribed for people with known coronary artery disease who want to reverse the disease in their clogged and damaged coronary arteries. Some people who are at high risk follow it to try to prevent coronary artery disease. This diet recommends that only 10 percent of calories come from fat. None of this fat is to come from cooking oils or animal products (except for nonfat milk and nonfat yogurt). This diet excludes fish. It excludes plant products high in fat such as avocados, nuts, and seeds. It is a diet high in fiber that allows moderate salt, sugar, and alcohol. While there is no calorie restriction, following it results in a low-calorie diet. This diet can lower blood pressure and cholesterol.

While this is a healthy diet that does reduce cardiac risk factors, it is a difficult one for most Americans to follow because of its extremely low fat content and strictly vegetarian nature. This diet, like all fad diets, banishes whole food groups—in this case, meats, poultry, fish, nuts, seeds, certain fats, and certain vegetables. These items are very good for you if taken in moderation. You do not need to be as strict with yourself as this diet leads you to believe. Its principles are sound, but its highly restrictive nature can make it difficult to stick with. A more moderate version will benefit you greatly. Try to eat lower-fat foods and more fruits and vegetables, watch your total calories (but include low-fat meats, fish, and poultry), and keep your fats unsaturated.

The Glycemic Index

Dr. David Jenkins at the University of Toronto developed this diet in 1981. His purpose was to try to find a diet for diabetes that could replace the complicated system of dietary exchanges diabetics have used for years to control their blood sugars. Diabetic exchanges are foods that are grouped according to similar calorie, carbohydrate, protein, and fat content. The exchange groups are starch / bread, meat, vegetables, fruit, milk, and fat. A person is allowed a certain number of exchange choices from each food list per meal per day. By eating from combinations of all food groups at meals, blood sugar is stabilized and controlled. The Glycemic Index (GI) ranks foods by how quickly they raise blood sugar. Foods with high Glycemic Index numbers (over 70) cause a quick spike in blood sugar, while foods with low Glycemic Index numbers (55 and below) break down more slowly. This diet ranks carbohydrates only, as proteins and fats don't cause the blood sugar to rise much.

The idea behind weight loss using the Glycemic Index is to eat more foods with a low Glycemic Index and fewer foods with a high Index. The theory is that by eating foods that do not raise your blood sugar much, you will minimize your body's release of insulin. Since insulin increases the storage of fat in the body, decreasing the amount of insulin released will decrease stored body fat. According to the theory, it will also decrease hunger, which is caused by the low blood sugar that results from the rapid removal of high blood sugar by the insulin. (This is complicated chemistry.) The idea is that high-glycemic diets may increase appetite, increase food intake, increase fat deposition, and overwork the cells that produce insulin.

There does seem to be merit to using the Glycemic Index for diabetics (although the American Diabetes Association has not adopted it as of this writing). Also, it may be useful for endurance athletes who need to be able to regulate carbohydrates for energy, sometimes wanting slow-sugar-release foods and sometimes wanting quick-sugar-release foods. The diet's role in weight loss has not been firmly proven as of this writing, although there are many studies under way.

The drawback to this diet is that the Index is only for individual foods, not foods in combination, and that may change a food's properties. Take, for example, a peanut butter and jelly sandwich: the jelly would have a high GI score, but when combined with the bread and peanut butter, the total GI score would be lower. The other drawback is that some foods with low GI scores are high in fat like peanuts or cashews for example. So following a diet plan based only on the Glycemic Index may increase your risk of heart attack and stroke. If you are diabetic, an endurance athlete, or simply interested in the role of sugar and insulin in the body, you may want to learn more about this nutritional theory, which is still being studied.

Extreme Low-Calorie Diets

Studies have shown that extreme low-calorie diets consisting of about two-thirds of the normally recommended daily calories result in significant lowering of most cardiovascular risk factors. Because they require such extreme calorie reduction there are no fad diets currently promoting them.

People who voluntarily followed these diets for six years significantly reduced their cholesterol levels, blood pressure, and other major risk factors for heart disease, along with risk factors for diabetes, cancer, and Alzheimer's. It is suspected that this lowering of both risk factors and body mass will lead to a longer life expectancy because the aging process is slowed.

This kind of diet requires careful medical supervision to ensure that the body obtains the necessary nutrients, which is difficult with such severe calorie restrictions. The diet usually consists of mostly complex carbohydrates from foods such as fruits and vegetables. This is not a diet for most to follow because it requires such intense discipline and restraint for one's whole life. It does prove though, like the low-fat vegetarian Ornish diet, that restricting calories does indeed reduce risk factors for disease. Furthermore, it proves that excess weight and high-fat, high-calorie diets speed aging and hasten death.

The Mediterranean Diet

The Mediterranean Diet is increasing in popularity. Many of us have tired of the low-carb craze and are looking for a sensible and enjoyable way to eat that will not be harmful to us. The Mediterranean Diet seems to fit this bill. The Mediterranean Diet evolved along the Mediterranean Sea and incorporates foods available in that region along with the cultural preferences of its people. The diet uses heart-healthy olive oil as its primary fat and it is rich in grains (pasta and breads), along with tomatoes, onions, artichokes, eggplants, peas, lentils, chickpeas, and fruits. Protein comes from grilled or steamed chicken and seafood (as opposed to red meat). And a glass or two of red wine a day is part of the diet.

Following this diet along with being physically active and not smoking has shown to extend life and reduce both cardiovascular disease and cancer. It also helps reduce some of the risks of metabolic syndrome, including lowering weight, blood pressure, levels of blood glucose, insulin levels, cholesterol and triglyceride levels, and markers for inflammation like C-reactive protein and homocysteine levels.

This is a diet that puts health, food, and pleasure together again and is best enjoyed in a leisurely way in the company of congenial companions. And it is not the only healthy regional diet in the world you can enjoy.

Cuisines from around the world have nourished humans in nutritionally sound ways for many thousands of years. Exploring the native foods of India, China, Japan, and others, so long as they are not adulterated with America's high-fat and high-sodium additions, can offer a variety of healthy and pleasurable ways of eating very different from the drive-through or packaged food choices that are most available to us in America. We can learn from our neighbors from around the world and our own Native American citizens—none of whom began struggling with obesity and all its attendant health problems until they abandoned their native dietary cultures and adopted our American way of eating. Now there is some food for thought.

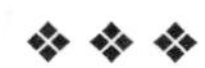

Nutrition Is Not a Diet

You may find a diet above that suits your temperament. You may not. Many of us need the requisite joys of eating to be a part of any plan we undertake. Food is a part of culture, family, hearth, and home. To remove that from the equation creates dissatisfaction in most people. This is one reason why diets invariably fail.

Nutrition is not a diet. Nor should you consider a nutritious way of eating as going on a diet. Nutrition means taking nourishment from food for the working of our bodies. Our diet is what and how much we eat, and determines whether our nutritional state is good or bad. In fact, diet simply means what we eat and drink. That is all. The word itself is not restrictive, nor does it imply any special selection of foods or drinks. A diet that supplies optimal nutrition for the body is a healthy diet. Weight loss comes when good sense is applied to feeding the body what it needs.

You can achieve lasting weight loss with just your common sense and sense of humor. Learn about nutritious foods. Follow the food groups. Manage your calorie load. Exercise more. Have fun. Finding joy in the possibilities of a healthy diet will carry you much further than complaining about what you "can't" have. Stick to it long enough, and you will come to realize that you no longer want what you "can't" have.

Eat healthy foods instead.

Eat foods that are minimally processed and fresh. If you eat more fruits and vegetables and less fats and salt, you'll probably be eating well. Drink an extra glass of water every day. Don't skip meals.

Don't deprive yourself of foods you like to eat.

If you will stick to healthy, fresh, unprocessed foods six days a week, indulging in your favorite other foods on the seventh will not harm you.

Eat six small, healthy meals a day.

This will result in more successful weight loss than three larger meals. The frequency of these meals prevents hunger that can provoke impulse eating and poor food choices.

Reduce portion sizes.

Portions that are too large, second helpings, and high-calorie snacks all contribute to weight gain. Some people have achieved remarkable weight loss simply by reducing their portion sizes with no other changes to diet or exercise.

Eliminate one soda or beer a day.

You could lose 10 pounds over the course of a year.

Figure out substitutions that work for you.

Trade high-fat foods for lower-fat alternatives that you like. Look for ways to lower fat. Eat frozen yogurt instead of ice cream. Use fat-free mayonnaise instead of regular, or trade the mayo for mustard, which is lower in fat. Drink 1 percent milk. Use cooking spray instead of oil. Avoid fast food (it's mostly fat and salt). Learn to cook using less fat.

Eat your meals slowly.

> *It takes 20 minutes for the brain to get the message that the body is full. Chew your food well, enjoy the taste, put your fork down in between bites, and think about and relish the food you are eating.*

Even though it seems we are all on a diet all the time, the fact is most of us are eating all the time. While our society idealizes and publicizes underweight models, it sells us high-fat fast food. We eat absolutely everywhere and all the time. We eat while watching television, we eat while at work at our desks, we eat when we shop, we eat when we go to sporting events, we eat at movies, we eat in our cars, and a lot of us probably eat in bed, too. Most of that eating is in addition to our regular meals. And most of that eating is not nutritionally sound.

Our nutritional state affects us in every way—from our mental and physical performance, to our sense of well-being, to our resistance (or susceptibility) to illness. When we are well-nourished, our bodies function optimally. Our weight is what it should be, and we have an adequate supply of carbohydrates, proteins, fats, vitamins, minerals, and water for our bodies to grow, repair damage, and fight off disease. We have adequate energy to accomplish the mental and physical activities we set out to perform. And we enjoy a sense of well-being that makes us feel at home in our bodies—balanced and comfortable.

> *Weight management is critical to health. But good nutrition is more than just weight management. Good nutrition means consuming the types of foods that our bodies need to do their work and fight off chronic disease.*

Good nutrition can be boiled down to one simple precept: *Eat a wide variety of whole foods.* In this world of fast foods, frozen foods, and convenience foods, what, you may ask, is a whole food? It is simply a food that is as *close to its natural state as possible.* It is a food that is not processed or refined, or only minimally so. It is a food grown in fertile soil or raised under natural conditions and consumed in its natural state. It is not treated with chemicals, processed by heat or irradiation, or genetically altered. It is a food prepared simply.

Examples of whole foods are fresh fruits and vegetables rather than those frozen, canned, or prepared with added ingredients; whole-wheat breads rather than those made from refined flour; whole grains such as brown rice rather than white; meat, poultry, or fish from a butcher or fishmonger rather than processed and treated foods such as deli meats, frozen fish sticks, or meats that come in a box.

The difference between whole foods and highly processed foods is that whole foods contain enzymes and other factors necessary for the proper, effective digestion and good assimilation of the nutrients nature has put into each particular food. Processed foods lose some of these natural factors and enzymes.

Studies have confirmed that eating more whole grains, legumes, fruits, vegetables, nuts, and seeds in their natural state helps to protect against cancer. It has been proven that diets high in refined white flour and white sugar lead to increased incidence of diabetes and dental cavities. Cultures whose diets consist primarily of natural foods that are not highly processed have much lower incidences of the chronic diseases than we suffer in this country.

The fact of the matter is that our knowledge of the precise effects of foods and food combinations is still incomplete. The biochemistry of good nutrition is very complex. At this point in our scientific knowledge, it is impossible to describe the "perfect" diet for each individual.

You can achieve a healthy and nutritious diet if you do the following:

- Eat a wide variety of whole foods.
- Reduce your consumption of processed and prepared foods from the supermarkets or fast food outlets.
- Reduce your portion sizes of meat, poultry, and fish.
- Increase your consumption of a variety of whole grains, fruits, and vegetables.
- Reduce your consumption of soft drinks and alcohol.
- Increase your consumption of fruit juices and water.

To begin the process of managing your weight with nutrition, learn about your food so you can make better choices to bring your body back into balance. Remember, the formula for weight loss is simple: *fewer calories, smarter choices,* and *more activity*.

Food Diary

Counting calories can be a pain, but it is less of a pain than wiping out entire food groups. And far, far healthier. You won't know what you are really eating until you actually measure and count.

For every 3,500 calories you are under your basic caloric need, you will lose one pound. Thus, if you decrease your food consumption by 500 calories a day, you may lose a pound a week (500 calories x 7 days = 3500 calories / week). Note: Some people find it easier to calculate calories by the week rather than by the day.

Learn to keep track of how much you are taking in. Also learn which foods have the most calories. For example, 1 gram of fat has 9 calories, while 1 gram of carbohydrate or protein has 4 calories. A whole baked potato may have only 200 calories, but just 1 tablespoon of butter adds 100 calories.

Your current body size, activity level, and metabolic rate determine how many calories you need per day to either lose or maintain your current weight. A calorie plan that is simple to follow is to allow 10 calories per pound of your ideal body weight. For example, if your ideal body weight is 150 pounds, your goal is to consume no more than 1,500 calories per day. If you stick to this amount of food intake, you will experience sustained weight loss.

If you want to maintain your weight, allow 15 calories per pound of your desired weight (as long as you are also getting a reasonable amount of exercise). To maintain your weight at 150 pounds, your goal is to consume no more than 2,250 calories per day. But if you are not exercising or have a slow metabolic rate, you may require fewer calories than this to avoid weight gain

To count your calorie intake and learn the nutritional content of the foods you eat, you need an easy-to-use nutrition guide and calorie counter. You can find such nutrition guides in bookstores, libraries, and software programs, and online. The U.S. Department of Agriculture (USDA) offers a searchable online nutrient database. That website is listed under Resources at the end of this book. Find a nutrition guide you like and that is easy to use. It should include (at least):

- Serving size
- Number of calories per serving

- Fat grams
- Sodium milligrams
- Cholesterol milligrams
- Carbohydrate grams
- Fiber grams

A blank food diary form is located in the Appendix. You can make copies to use to help analyze your food intake for a few weeks.

You will need to know the weight or portion size of the food you are eating to accurately count calories. Use a food scale, or estimate portion sizes to track your food consumption. Measuring is the best way to learn the calories and nutrients you are taking in. If you are estimating your serving sizes, consider a portion the size of a tennis ball to be approximately 1 cup and compare meat portions to a deck of cards. A portion of meat the size of a deck of cards is approximately 3 ounces. (Keep a tennis ball and a deck of cards in the kitchen while you are keeping your diary if you use this method so you won't over- or under-estimate.) Measuring liquids in a measuring cup is easy to do. Remember, if your measurement is wrong, your calorie counts will be wrong, too, and you won't find out what you want to know.

Record everything you eat and drink. If you have never kept a food diary, keeping a detailed one for a few weeks will be an eye-opening experience. The USDA recommends the following for good nutrition. Your food diary should help you determine which food groups you habitually ignore and allow you to bring them back into your diet.

Bread, Cereal, Rice, and Pasta Group (Grains Group)—whole grain and refined

(6 servings each equivalent to 1 ounce recommended per day)

- 1 slice of bread
- About 1 cup of ready-to-eat cereal flakes
- ½ cup of cooked cereal, rice, or pasta

Fruit Group

(4 servings or 2 cups recommended per day)

- 1 medium apple, banana, orange, pear
- ½ cup of chopped, cooked, or canned fruit

- ¾ cup of fruit juice

Vegetable Group

(5 servings or 2½ cups recommended per day)

- 1 cup of raw leafy vegetables
- ½ cup of other vegetables—cooked or raw
- ¾ cup of vegetable juice
- Dry beans, peas, and lentils can be counted as servings in either the meat and beans group or the vegetable group. If counted as a vegetable, the serving size is ½ cup as well.

Milk, Yogurt, and Cheese Group (Dairy Group)

(3 servings or 3 cups of low- fat or fat-free dairy recommended per day)

- 1 cup of milk or yogurt (includes lactose-free dairy)
- 1½ ounces of natural cheese (choose reduced-fat or fat-free most often)
- 2 ounces of processed cheese (such as American)
- 1 cup of soy-based beverage with added calcium

Meat, Poultry, Fish, Dry Beans, Eggs, and Nuts Group (Protein Group)

(5.5 ounces recommended per day—a 3-ounce serving is about the size of a deck of cards)

- 2–3 ounces of cooked lean meat, poultry, or fish
- ½ cup of cooked dry beans or ½ cup of tofu counts as 1 ounce of lean meat
- 2½-ounce soy burger or 1 egg counts as 1 ounce of lean meat
- 2 tablespoons of peanut butter or ⅓ cup of nuts

Note: Many of the serving sizes given above are smaller than those on the Nutrition Facts Label that appears on the back of a food item you buy in the store. For example, 1 serving of cooked cereal, rice, or pasta is 1 cup on a food label, but only ½ cup for the pyramid. This can lead to problems with your calorie counts if you do not pay attention.

Know How to Read a Food Label

Food labeling to prohibit untrue claims on packages and protect consumers was enacted in 1924 under the Federal Food and Drug Act. It has been under the jurisdiction of the Food and Drug Administration (FDA) and the U.S. Department of Agriculture (USDA) since then. In 1994, the current food label (shown here) was introduced to assist consumers in making healthier food choices by knowing the nutritional content of packaged foods. The current food label contains the following information:

- **Serving Size:** All the amounts that follow on the label are based on the serving size.
- **Servings Per Container:** *When you look at calories, fat, sodium, etc., you have to multiply them by the Servings Per Container* to know how much of each is in that package or can. This is tricky, so don't be fooled. For example, you buy a frozen food and even though the label says there are four servings in the package, you and I (and the manufacturer) all know that you are going to eat the whole thing. To figure out what's in that food package then, you must multiply times four the calories, fat grams, and all the other numbers to know what you are actually taking in. Don't be fooled by labels that have low calories, low fat, or low sodium, but multiple servings per container. You will get the hang of this after you read labels for a while.

Nutrition Facts/
Datos De Nutrición

Serving Size/Tamaño por Ración: 1 Package/Paquete (354 g)
Servings Per Container/Raciones por Envase: 1

Amount Per Serving/Cantidad por Ración	
Calories/Calorías 270 Calories from Fat/Calorías de Grasa 70	
	% Daily Value*/% Valor Diario*
Total Fat/Grasa Total 8 g	**13%**
Saturated Fat/Grasa Saturada 4 g	**20%**
Trans Fat/Grasa Trans 0 g	
Polyunsaturated Fat/Grasa Poliinsaturada .5 g	
Monounsaturated Fat/Grasa Monoinsaturada 3 g	
Cholesterol/Colesterol 45 mg	**15%**
Sodium/Sodio 650 mg	**27%**
Potassium/Potasio 950 mg	**27%**
Total Carbohydrate/Carbohidrato Total 27 g	**9%**
Dietary Fiber/Fibra Dietética 10 g	**40%**
Sugars/Azúcares 10 g	
Protein/Proteínas 22 g	

Vitamin/Vitamina A 90% • Vitamin/Vitamina C 0%
Calcium/Calcio 10% • Iron/Hierro 15%

*Percent Daily Values are based on a 2,000 calorie diet. Your daily values may be higher or lower depending on your calorie needs:
*Los porcentajes de Valores Diarios están basados en una dieta de 2,000 calorías. Sus valores diarios pueden ser mayores o menores dependiendo de sus necesidades calóricas:

	Calories/Calorías	2,000	2,500
Total Fat/Grasa Total	Less than/Menos que	65g	80g
Sat. Fat/Grasa Sat.	Less than/Menos que	20g	25g
Cholesterol/Colesterol	Less than/Menos que	300mg	300mg
Sodium/Sodio	Less than/Menos que	2,400mg	2,400mg
Potassium/Potasio	Less than/Menos que	3,500mg	3,500mg
Total Carbohydrate/Carbohidrato Total		300g	375g
Dietary Fiber/Fibra Dietética		25g	30g

Some labels, like the one shown above, have the information in two languages

- **Calories:** The food label will give you the number of *calories per serving,* so don't forget to calculate how much of the package you are going to eat to see how many calories you are taking in. Reading our sample food label, if you eat half the package you are taking in 135 calories; if you eat the whole thing, you are taking in 270 calories. The label also gives you the number of calories from fat. This will tell you whether this is a low-fat or a high-fat food. Foods that are less than 30 percent fat are considered low-fat. This example would be considered a low-fat food because it is less than 30 percent fat. (Thirty calories from fat is 1/3 or 30 percent of the total 270 calories per serving. If this food had 140 calories from fat, that would make it more than 50 percent fat—140 calories is more than half the total 270 calories per serving, therefore, that would be a high-fat food.)

- **Total Fat:** This gives both the total fat grams and the saturated fat grams. Fat is part of most foods. We need to eat some fat to maintain good health. What makes eating fat somewhat complicated is that different types of fats have different effects on health—especially heart health.

  Saturated Fats tend to raise blood cholesterol. These foods include high-fat dairy products (like cheese, whole milk, cream, butter, and regular ice cream), fatty fresh and processed meats, the skin and fat of poultry, lard, palm oil, and coconut oil. Keep your intake of these foods low (less than 10 percent of your total daily calories). Trans fats, though unsaturated, also raise cholesterol.

  Unsaturated Fats do not raise blood cholesterol. Unsaturated fats occur in vegetable oils, most nuts, olives, avocados, and fatty fish like salmon. Unsaturated oils include both monounsaturated fats and polyunsaturated fats. Olive, canola, sunflower, and peanut oils are some of the oils high in monounsaturated fats. Vegetable oils such as soybean, corn, and cottonseed and many kinds of nuts are good sources of polyunsaturated fats. Some fish, such as salmon, tuna, and mackerel, contain omega-3 fatty acids. Omega-3 fatty acids are fats that protect against heart disease and stroke, lower cholesterol, and even alleviate arthritis. Unsaturated fats, including omega-3s, are the good fats. Use moderate amounts of food high in unsaturated fats, taking care to avoid excess calories.

  Total fat should be kept between 20 percent to 35 percent of your total calories per day for adults (25 percent to 40 percent for children). Saturated fat and trans fat should be limited in everyone's diet because it contributes to high cholesterol and heart disease. Fat has 9 calories per gram.

- **Cholesterol:** Remember that cholesterol is a fat (both in foods and in the body), so reducing your dietary fat will also reduce your dietary cholesterol. Dietary cholesterol is found in food products derived from animals (the highest cholesterol foods are liver and other organ meats, egg yolks, and dairy fats). Dietary cholesterol is not present in grains, fruits, or vegetables. Try to keep your dietary cholesterol intake under 300 mg per day, remembering that your body makes cholesterol, too. If cholesterol is high in your blood, you want to decrease the amount of cholesterol in your diet.
- **Sodium:** The recommended amount of sodium per day is 2,300 mg. This is equivalent to 1 level teaspoon of table salt per day. In fact, we only need ¼ of a teaspoon for our body's health. Simply put: most Americans get too much salt in their diet because of the high proportion of prepared foods they consume. By reading food labels, you will learn which foods are high in sodium. Remember to consider the amount of sodium in a particular food in relation to the amount of sodium you are consuming the rest of the day in other foods.
- **Total Carbohydrates:** This gives you the number of grams of carbohydrates. These come from the grains, fruits, and vegetable food groups, as well as sweets. The body turns all carbohydrates into glucose that it burns as fuel. There are two types of carbohydrates: complex and simple. Simple carbohydrates are sugars; complex carbohydrates are starches. In addition to supplying energy, complex carbs (carbohydrates) contain vitamins, minerals, and fiber. It is recommended that 45 percent to 65 percent of your diet consist of complex carbohydrates. Both complex and simple carbs are found in fruits, vegetables, legumes, and grains. Sweets and refined carbs (like sugar and white flour) lack vitamins, minerals, and fiber and are high in calories. These are the carbs that should be limited in the diet. Complex carbs provide energy, fiber, and nutrients and are required for good nutrition. There are 4 calories per gram for both simple and complex carbohydrates. To calculate the number of calories from carbs, multiply the number of grams by four.
- **Dietary Fiber:** A high-fiber diet has many health benefits. It is believed to lower the risk of colon cancer; it prevents and treats constipation; it can regulate and control troubling conditions like

irritable bowel syndrome; it may help control blood sugar in diabetics; and it lowers cholesterol, too. It is also filling, so it helps decrease hunger. Fiber is found in whole grains, fruits, and vegetables. It is recommended that women get between 20 and 25 grams of fiber a day and men between 30 and 40 grams. Foods with the highest fiber are fruits and vegetables with edible skins and whole-grain cereals.

- **Sugars:** A diet high in sugar is a diet high in calories but low in nutrients. High sugar consumption can provoke or worsen diabetes, cause dental cavities, and contribute to obesity. There are two types of sugars. Simple sugars are naturally occurring and are the sweets in fruits and the starches in vegetables. Refined sugars are those that have been processed to remove their vitamins, minerals, and fiber, thus causing them to lose their nutritional value. Refined sugars include white sugar, white flour, and processed foods. Refined sugars in the diet cause sugar in the blood to rise and insulin to be released from the pancreas. Insulin in the blood causes fat to be formed instead of burned. Refined sugars cause insulin to rise more than simple sugars do, so it is important to limit your intake of refined sugars. If you are diabetic or overweight, you will need to monitor your sugar intake carefully.
- **Protein:** This gives you the number of grams of protein. Protein content is highest in meats, chicken, fish, milk products, and eggs. It is necessary to the body for tissue growth and repair. It is recommended that between 10 percent to 35 percent of your diet consist of proteins. Pregnant women need the highest amount for growth of the unborn baby. There are 4 calories per gram for protein, so to calculate the percentage of calories from protein, multiply the number of grams by four.
- **Vitamin A, Vitamin C, Calcium, Iron:** These are listed on the Food Label to give you an idea of how much of your daily requirement a particular food provides. A healthy diet is composed of dozens of nutrients, all of which could not be listed, so these are chosen. They are not necessarily the most important, but calcium and iron are two that some people should watch.

  Calcium: This nutrient must be present to build strong bones and teeth. It is very important in childhood during growth and for women at risk for osteoporosis. Children who drink too many soft drinks and not enough milk are at risk of deficiency, particularly girls. During their teens, girls begin "banking" calcium in their bones that will later help prevent fractures and spinal deformity when they reach their 70s. You should get 1,200 to 1,500 mg of calcium a day through your diet. Add supplements if necessary.

Iron: This nutrient is necessary to build healthy blood cells. Blood cells live about 120 days, so you need a constant supply of iron to keep making them. If you are deficient in it, you may suffer iron-deficiency anemia. Vegetarians and women who are menstruating are at risk for iron deficiency.

- **Percent Daily Values:** This last part of the Food Label does some calculations for you to give you an idea of what your daily totals should be for Fat, Cholesterol, Sodium, and Carbohydrates based on a 2,000- and 2,500-calorie per day diet.

The simple truth is, most of us get too few fruits and vegetables, too many calories, and too much fat in our daily diets. While it seems to make sense to just take vitamins to make up for the nutrients we are missing, that hasn't yet been proven to work. So far, the science finds more protection coming from the foods themselves—like fruits and vegetables—than from supplements.

Bringing good nutrition into our lives is a robust expression of balance. It reconnects us to our human experience by making our food a sacred part of life. Consuming the freshest and most natural foods serves to remind us that we are part of a larger whole and that health is our natural state of grace. There is no such thing as a food that is new and improved over the classic version offered by Mother Nature. Apply what you have learned here and discover how natural whole food is the fuel that stokes the furnace of good health.

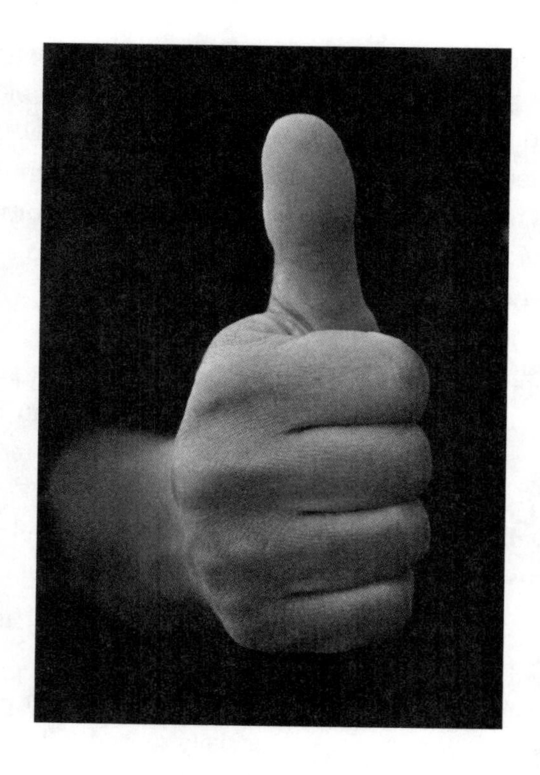

Your Third Choice: *Mental Resilience*

Here is a choice that will carry you across the threshold and deliver you to your ultimate destination—a place of true peace, happiness, and self-acceptance.

You may not see a change in your body shape—but it will change your body image. It may not change the landscape of your life—but it will change how you cultivate that land. This choice is about enriching the health of your mind and spirit.

> *As the pilot of your body, the mind is more powerful than most give it credit for. A flexible mind is a resilient one. And a resilient mind can carry you through dark times, stormy nights, and emotional whirlwinds.*

Mental resilience is the quality that will allow you to master your health risks, succeed at behavioral change, and live a happy and satisfying life. There are few qualities more necessary to living well and cultivating good health than resilience. Mental resilience means hardiness of the mind and spirit. It is a collection of strategies you always have available to you. It enables you to remain hopeful in the face of adversity and to trust in your ability to recover from and prevail over setbacks, disappointments, grief, and loss.

This ability is a hallmark of great leaders and world champions. These remarkable individuals seem to draw from a never-ending source within themselves. Their emotional strength and power rise in proportion to the challenges they face, so they always seem equal to the task before them, no matter how challenging. This can be you.

While some seem to be born with mental resilience, for most people, it grows. Mental resilience is most often learned. You can cultivate it in your own life starting today. If you feel overwhelmed and helpless in the face of life's challenges, you can find ways to increase your share of joy and satisfaction. Many creative activities foster mental resilience. Many spiritual beliefs strengthen and support this resilience. Focusing on these productive, positive modes of thinking can gradually extinguish destructive behaviors and attitudes. That is why creating and owning your mental experience can be such a powerful weapon for all-around health.

All humans have a spiritual nature. Our spirit expresses itself through action, purpose, and emotion. Being in touch with and in harmony with this spirit is achieved by cultivating an inner life that gives you strength, provides comfort, and enables you to bear the unbearable. Spirituality means having faith. It means believing that there is rarely anything given to you that you cannot handle.

People live and wear their spirituality in many different ways. The world's major religions are testaments to our human need for a spiritual life. While some find their spiritual expression through religion, others find it in different ways, such as philosophy, meditation, art, music, or time spent with nature. However your spirituality expresses itself, honoring and nurturing it will enhance your mental resilience and give your life added meaning. And meaning is like water to the soul.

Through spirituality and personal examination, you can find your purpose in the world. When your life has meaning and you have found your purpose, the shallow distractions of life lose their power over you. Your purpose fills your days with positive direction. It becomes something that is part of you, something you know without the need for question. It gives you such a strong foundation that you are able to deal with whatever life throws at you. That is when you know you have found real resilience.

Sometimes the roller coaster of emotion keeps you from finding your inner strength. Emotions are like lenses through which you see and experience life. If you cannot see through them, sense them coming, and understand their impact on your state of mind, you will always find yourself tossed about on their stormy seas. You may freeze up in an effort to avoid these feelings. Avoiding your feelings wreaks havoc on your ability to deal with the difficulties in life.

But emotions are transient—they come and go. Mental resilience comes with being able to ride the waves of strong emotions. Learning balance is as important to your emotional life as it is to other aspects of living. By trusting in balance you can experience all emotions with grace, even the truly unpleasant ones, knowing the pendulum will always swing back toward the center. If you can avoid obsessive thinking about things that worry or anger you while maintaining a focus on the positive aspects of your life, your ability to balance your emotions will lead to a strong mental resilience.

Being able to experience and express your feelings helps relieve the pressures of simply being alive. Recognizing your emotional states and understanding the causes of your emotions will give you greater self-knowledge and control over your inner life. Use your emotions to learn who you are and what is important to you. Then use this understanding to navigate through your life with poise and grace. Your inner strength and comfort will not only lead you to greater happiness, but it will draw helpful people to you, too.

We humans are social creatures. Nothing erodes mental resilience more than isolation. That's why solitary confinement is the worst punishment that can be inflicted on a prisoner. Isolation is also a characteristic of mental illness. Human connections and belonging are as essential for health and happiness as level emotions and spirituality. They all feed one another. Keep yourself connected.

The family is the fundamental unit of human belonging. The ability to form connections grows out of this primary unit. However, if the family to which you were born is unable to meet your relationship needs, it is still possible to establish productive human relationships at any time and at any age. What we all need is trust, commitment, and connection. We long to love and to feel loved. Being able to spend time with, give to, and do things for others protects us from isolation and enriches our lives.

From the individual outward to the family, the village, the nation, and the world, we are all connected and we all belong to each other. Keeping personal connections strong and healthy builds individual strength. Developing intimate relationships is known to improve health and extend life. The act of intimacy, the ability to share one's essential, innermost, deepest nature with another, keeps the emotional gates open. It reassures us that what we are feeling and experiencing is not ours alone. It creates a network of trust that supports and nourishes us as we move through our lives.

If you are lucky, you will enjoy meaningful and healthy relationships with many people in your life. Your family, your spouse, your friends, the colleagues with whom you work, and larger social networks all provide possibilities to forge this necessary human connection. It is your connection to yourself and others that allows you to find the full range of your strength.

But even with all the resilience in the world, life is sometimes heartbreaking. Everyone will suffer frustration, unfairness, disappointment, setbacks, or grief at one time or another. It is the human condition. Sometimes the greatest expression of your resilience is simply making it through each day and waiting for the clouds to pass. If you manage to pass through your period of darkness with patience and take comfort in some simple human experiences, you are operating out of healthy mental resilience.

Something as simple as just getting up in the morning, having a nice breakfast, and going for a walk may help you get through the day. Watching children play, planting a garden, and listening to music all comfort the soul.

A walk in the woods, swimming in the ocean, hiking up a mountain, watching a sunrise or a sunset are all activities that can return you to your source and help you through the difficulties. Visiting with friends and having a laugh helps to remind you that life moves on and that you can move with it. A sense of humor is essential—it is resilience at its most humble and its very finest.

Be authentic to yourself. Allow yourself to rest. Allow yourself to appreciate completion of goals. Understand that your thoughts, attitudes, and self-talk are powerful determinants of your health. Seek positive relationships. Laugh as much as possible. Seek satisfaction instead of perfection.

When you harness mental resilience, you will discover that you can meet whatever comes with courage, optimism, and faith. In the end, that's all you can ask of yourself and the best you can do.

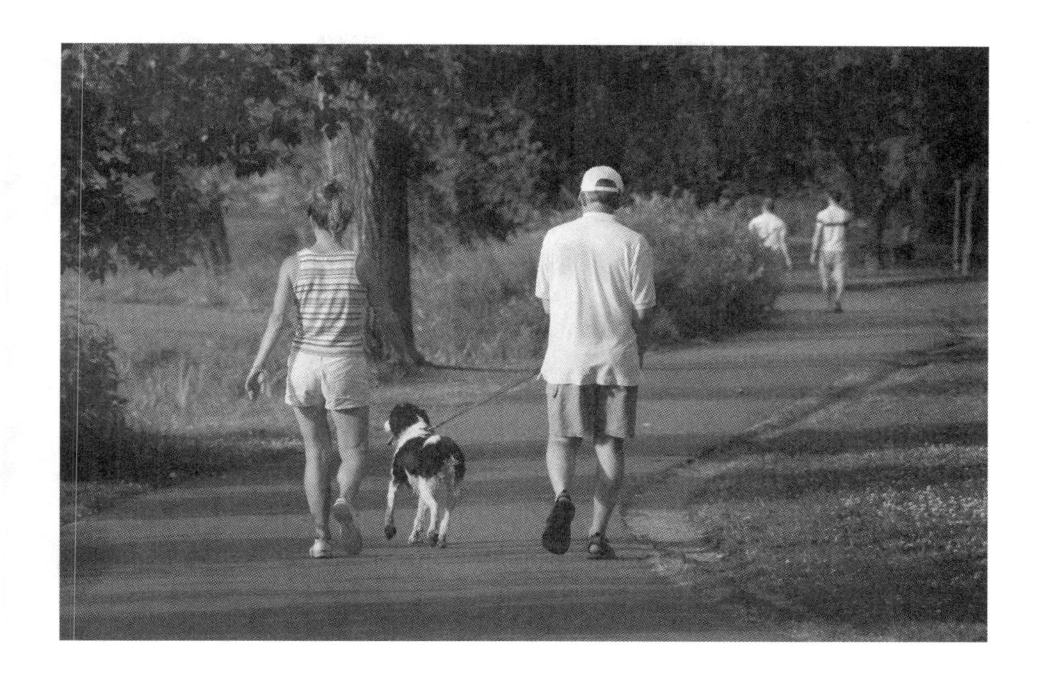

Change: *How to Stick with Your Choices*

Now you know your health risks. Congratulations, that's half the battle. And you know the behaviors that will reduce your risks. Here's where the rubber meets the road—you are going to try to improve your health by changing any of your behaviors that are harming it.

So, how do you change? First, create a picture in your mind of how you want your life and your health to be better. You have just taken the first step.

Are you thinking about changing a behavior or two to reduce your health risks? That's a great idea! If you will aim your behavior changes at achieving specific goals, you can successfully reduce most of your controllable health risks. In the process you will move yourself onto a path of improved health, happiness, and longevity.

The behavior changes you choose may be as simple as taking your medication properly or as hard as losing weight, beginning an exercise program, or quitting smoking. It all depends on your particular health risks and what you want to do about them. You may just need to fine-tune a few things you're already doing, or you may need to completely overhaul your current lifestyle. Either way you are encouraged to start small, go slow, and never lose sight of the goals you are trying to reach. *They are finite and measurable.* The process can feel overwhelming, but if you know where you're headed, all you really have to do is put one foot in front of the other and let time do the rest. So, before we discuss how to change, let's first talk about the change process itself—specifically the behavior change process.

Change *is* a process. If you familiarize yourself with how the process works, you will improve your chances of success because your knowledge will help you prepare for the changes you are planning to make.

Let's be honest, if change were easy, this book would only be 10 pages long. Change can be difficult, even downright scary. But the good news is that once you have a firm handle on where you are going and why, change becomes easier. Take your time, add some patience, and the change will integrate itself into your life. One day you will wonder that it seemed difficult at all.

The simple secret to mastering behavioral change is to understand the following change equation:

Knowledge + Desire + Time = Change

Knowledge is powerful. You cannot "unknow" what you know. Once you know your health risks, you will not be able to forget what you have learned. Knowledge is what gives you the power to change. Knowledge will lead to change when you add desire to the equation.

Desire is born of this knowledge. You cannot desire what you do not know. Knowledge plus desire is remarkably powerful. The discipline you need for change will come when you focus your attention on fulfilling your desires. When you focus on your desires, your body and emotions will gravitate toward fulfilling whatever it is that you desire.

Finally, time is the fairy dust of change. It is your ally and your friend. Work with it and not against it, and you will have a powerful weapon in your will-power arsenal.

When knowledge, desire, and time join together, they can inspire a complete behavioral transformation. Allow them to help remove the barriers of competing interests and habits that jockey for your attention. It is natural to invest your time in the things that are important to you, but, sadly, most of us don't appreciate the importance of our health until we lose it. Don't let that be you.

> *Your health is the most important asset you own. Are you doing everything you can to protect it?*

So how do you begin?

> *First, you must* ***want*** *to change more than you want the status quo. If you don't, you won't be successful. Only you can decide how important your health is and what you are willing to do to preserve it.*

Clear and straightforward steps are offered here, but you must choose to take them. And in taking them, you will leave your comfortable habit zone. But trust that this is a wonderful thing.

We humans are creatures of habit. We love our habits. They comfort us, make us feel safe, and give our lives a sense of stability. At the same time, our habits can be cages that imprison us and keep us from fulfilling our highest potential. The trick to making a healthy behavior change is to trade habits that are harming us for habits that make us healthier and happier.

Your goal is to grow new healthy habits to replace old unhealthy ones. Now that you have learned the hazards of unhealthy behaviors, perhaps the benefits of healthy ones have become more desirable. Once you establish them, good habits are just as comfortable as bad habits—if not more so. These new, better habits create the transformational change that leads to a healthier, longer life and a whole powerful new you. It's a rebirth you can experience any time, at any age.

Humans change in stages; everything doesn't happen at once. Your health provider can be a great partner and help guide you through the stages so you can keep moving forward with your change. It's not uncommon to get stuck in a certain stage or even to regress to an earlier stage when you're in the process of making a permanent behavior change.

This does not mean failure. It only means there are still lessons you are learning and tasks you have not yet mastered. Nothing of real value is ever offered up without a price to pay and that includes your health.

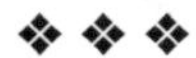

The Stages of Change

Precontemplation

You're not even thinking about making any changes. The only way to move on from this stage is to seek information and consider whether your life as it is now is everything you want it to be. Reading this book may be all you need to move on.

Contemplation

Now you are thinking about making a change. Maybe you're not ready to start today or even tomorrow, but you plan to make a change within the next six months. This is a great time to get out a piece of paper and make a list of the pros and cons of the health risks you've identified. List both the benefits from reducing them and the difficulties required to reduce them. See the questions below to get an idea of where you are and what you want to do about what you've learned.

Preparation

You are beyond just thinking about change, you're planning to make it happen anywhere within a month to six months. The best thing you can do at this stage is to choose clear and measurable goals—behaviors you are willing to commit to. Rather than say to yourself, "I'm going to exercise more." Say, "I am going to walk 240 minutes a week at my target heart rate." You can measure how many minutes you walk each week, and you can measure your heart rate when you do walk.

When you are preparing to make a change make sure of three things:

1. Your goal is a behavior.
2. The behavior can be measured.
3. It's a behavior you are confident you can stick to for 12 weeks.

For example, if a treadmill is boring to you, don't plan to spend four hours a week on it. You won't do it. Small changes over time yield bigger rewards than big changes you don't stick to. A good plan developed in the preparation stage will serve you well through the entire change process.

Action

This is where you're doing it! You get up every morning and recommit yourself to your change. You don't have to be perfect to succeed, just committed. This is the stage where you face your difficulties and impose your will in order to achieve the goals you want to reach. This is the stage where help is available if you need it. Alcoholics Anonymous, Weight Watchers, and Maverick's Smart Health Choices are all programs designed to help guide you through the Action phase of your change. Get through this stage and you are almost there.

Maintenance

You've done it! You've stuck to your chosen behaviors for 12 weeks, you've overcome your difficulties, you've held yourself accountable, and you've created new habits. The challenge of this stage is to keep right on with your new behaviors and avoid backsliding. It's the repetition of new habits that carves them into life patterns that make you uncomfortable when you give them up.

Termination

This is where your dream has come true! You have complete control of and total commitment to the new behavior. There are no inner struggles and you have no fear of relapse. You have made it.

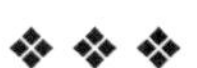

Beginning the Change

First, ask yourself the following questions (and write down the answers):

- What specifically about my health do I need to change and why?
- What habits are holding me back?
- What do I stand to lose if I don't change?
- What do I stand to gain if I do change?
- What am I willing to do to make the change happen?

Your answers will guide you in the right direction for you. They are the treasure map you will follow that will lead you to the treasure—control over your health and comfort in your life. They will help you stay true to the journey.

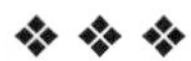

Develop the Will

The time is always right for you to undertake behavioral change. Just thinking about it has already begun to lay the groundwork. With a solid plan of attack, the changes you make will eventually seem to be the most natural and right thing in the world for you.

Having answered the questions above, you now know what it is about your health you want to change. You know what you are willing to do to make it happen. But now you need to set yourself up for success. The following are a few issues that, when resolved, will help to make your transition smoother and more comfortable. By having your mind set in this mode of right thinking, you will be better able to make successful health changes.

Keys to Success

Motivation: Are you highly motivated? Are you willing to do whatever it takes to make it happen?	❑ Yes	❑ No
Time: Have you made the time you need to implement your change? Are you willing to continue doing so?	❑ Yes	❑ No
Support: Do you have support lined up to help you? Do you have something or someone to offer encouragement or professional and personal support during your change?	❑ Yes	❑ No
Triggers: Have you identified "triggers" that can throw you back into old behaviors, and do you have a plan for avoiding them?	❑ Yes	❑ No
Goals: Do you have measurable goals so you will know when you are succeeding?	❑ Yes	❑ No

Answering *yes* to these questions will replace doubt with certainty. You will develop the positive ability to manage your plan. Remember, knowing is half the battle.

But nothing will happen until you take action.
Action is how you win the war.

This is the moment to transition from simple **Contemplation** to serious **Preparation.** You are beginning to desire making a positive change over the current situation. You are beginning to develop a plan and considering different ways to achieve it.

The next step will be putting your plan into **Action**. Making it happen.

And then **Maintenance**—keeping it alive by replacing old behaviors with new ones.

Your ultimate goal is **Termination**—that is the moment when you know beyond a shadow of a doubt that you own the change.

It's yours.

Be aware that change is cyclical, and a lapse from the plan does not mean failure. Continue to be kind to yourself. Do not believe that you have abandoned your commitment to change; relapse is not failure, but rather a cycle that you are moving through on the road to new habits. Look for the reasons behind the relapse. Then continue to seek the healthy change that you desire.

It is normal for you to feel a little uncomfortable when you first start to make a change, and you may want to give up at times. It is a natural human impulse to seek comfort and avoid discomfort. When undertaking change, it is necessary to remain focused on the healthful decision you have made. *If your desire for change is stronger than your discomfort, you will succeed.* The following will help you manage this discomfort more easily:

- **Be positive.** Life isn't fair and things rarely happen as they "should." But when you initiate a change, the more you control how you react and feel, the calmer you will be. Don't let events and circumstances dictate your actions and reactions.
- **Make the best of it.** Handle the situation that exists and don't waste time reflecting on the "shoulds." If you focus on results and don't get too preoccupied about how you feel about the change itself, it will be easier. Be as low key as necessary and stick with your plan.

- **Don't resist.** This is going to happen. Use this change to your advantage. The more you resist it, the more energy you will waste that could be spent in better ways. Use change to steer your life in the direction you want it to go.
- **Take responsibility.** Accept the results of the choices you make, be flexible; do good work. *Remember, no one owes you anything.* You create what you have and how you feel about it.
- **Think bigger.** Find something that will lift your spirits and energize you. Be of service to others. It will do more for you than you can imagine and help others at the same time. It will help you weather change and keep life in perspective.
- **Let your will be your ally.** It, too, knows what you want. Lay down this groundwork and make the change with humor and grace. Once you have started the wheel of change rolling, you must hold on and ride it with tenacity. If you are successful, these changes will land you on the shores of brand new possibilities.

Freedom in 12 Weeks

Once you have planned your change, there must be sufficient *time* for the new behaviors you undertake to become comfortable habits. **Twelve weeks is the best time frame for making change.**

Why 12 weeks? Because it is a short enough time to hang tough, but a long enough period so that you will see measurable results from your efforts. Whether your behavior change involves weight loss, exercise, blood pressure or blood sugar control, quitting smoking or drinking, if you can *hang tough* for 12 weeks, you *will* see change and you *will* get more comfortable with it, *guaranteed.*

At the end of this 12-week period, you will experience a sense of comfort with the new behavior. What was once strange, new, and a little uncomfortable is now familiar and habitual. You will need to continue to reinforce the behavior, of course, but that will be easier because it is what you now have become *used to.* A new habit has been born! The biggest mistake people make when trying to make behavioral change is not allowing adequate time for the change to take hold. They "short-change" themselves. At a certain point, you just have to show up every day, stick to your plan, and let time work its magic.

In the next 12 weeks, you will reach for goals that will reduce your risk of disease. As a bonus, you will prove to yourself that you can achieve any health goal you choose. Choosing goals and making a plan to reach them is the most effective way not only to enhance your health and prevent disease—but to build the life you want and achieve your most cherished dreams.

Steps to success

Follow these steps to successfully reach your chosen goals and, at the same time, see how well you can make behavioral change work for you:

- **Select your goals.** There may be just one goal you want to focus on or maybe there is more than one. The important thing is to pick the goals that are most relevant to your situation and / or ones that you are most eager to reach. Make a list of your risk factors and put a goal next to each one. Each goal you pick will likely reduce more than a single health risk.
- **Look at your calendar.** Decide where you want to be 12 weeks from now. Big goals may take longer than 12 weeks. For example, if you have a lot of weight to lose, make a 12-week plan to lose one pound per week. Once you have been successful with that, you will be able to lose all the weight you want as long as you have enough time. Remember, you are looking for new ways to live that improve your life and that you can enjoy each day.
- **Make a list of the behaviors that will accomplish your goal.** Now make a three-column list of Health Risks and Goals and the Behaviors that will achieve your goals. Behaviors are things you DO, not things you think about doing. For example, you may want to see your health practitioner for lab tests or medications. You may want to practice a new behavior like cooking in a more healthy way, doing yoga or meditation daily, etc. You may want to attend a class to learn more about a particular risk like diabetes. You may choose to *add* a new behavior to your life, like exercising daily or eating six small meals a

day instead of skipping certain meals and overeating at others. Or you may choose to *eliminate* a certain behavior, like smoking or drinking. *Be very specific. These are the behaviors you are committed to* **doing** *for the next 12 weeks. Commit to sticking to the behaviors you chose for 12 full weeks. Don't try to do too much. You should be confident you can complete the behaviors you choose.*

My Health Risks	My Goals	Behaviors to Reach Goals

- **Chart these behaviors on a monthly calendar for 12 weeks.** Write down the behaviors you are going to perform (or eliminate) for each day. Plan ahead for any events in your life or on your calendar in the coming 12 weeks that may challenge your change efforts and make a plan to work around them. Each day that you complete (or refrain from) your goal behavior, check it off your calendar or highlight it with colorful markers. Using highlighters or stickers on your calendar can be a surprisingly powerful incentive on days when you may feel like wavering. You may find that you will follow through with the behavior some days just so you will be able to check or highlight that you did it on your 12-week calendar.

- **You may take a day off every week if you need to**—*but no more than one.* If you adhere to your plan with dedication six days out of seven, you WILL succeed. Knowing you've got one free day every week helps keep you motivated and acts as a pressure valve to keep you from stopping your change prematurely. You will know the change you have chosen is a good one when you don't feel like abandoning it on your free day. In the meantime, remember your efforts are about making your life happier, healthier, and more in your control. A sense of freedom is essential to being a powerful and effective person, and a free day once a week gives you that freedom.

  Note: Free days do NOT apply to addictions like smoking, alcohol abuse, or eating disorders. The only way to conquer addiction is to stop the behavior COMPLETELY. The slightest relapse can undo all you have done and may require you to start all over from the beginning again. Relapse doesn't mean failure, but it can slow your progress and make a change that much harder. Free days also do not apply to safety goals like medication compliance, seatbelts, bike helmets, etc. Let your common sense guide you.

- **Be valiant.** There will be bumps in the road, points where old behaviors are still clinging hard. Change is cyclical, and a relapse to old behaviors does not equal failure. The greater your desire to reach a final outcome, the more likely you are to eventually achieve it, regardless of how many times you fail in the interim. Behavior change takes time. Changing behavior is hard. How hard it is and how long it will take is different for everybody. We all love our habits and we all tend to resist change. So, don't be too hard on yourself when you experience difficulty adjusting, but don't let yourself off the hook, either.

Start NOW!

This minute can be the beginning of your 12-week plan and a whole new and better life. Start *right now* by creating images in your mind of what you want to achieve. Imagine your life in a new and better place—visualize yourself feeling vibrant and whole, being physically, mentally, emotionally, and spiritually strong. That's your destination.

Ultimately nothing will happen that you don't make happen. Be resolute. Make healthy choices that you can live with and come to love. Be true to yourself. And start thinking of rewards for yourself that you will earn with your achievements.

Once you have settled on a plan, all that is left is to behave with unwavering devotion to it for 12 full weeks. It is the passage of time that will effect the change. If you will put your trust in that, you will experience change. *Do not decide on the goodness or badness of any change until you have adhered to it for 12 full weeks.*

Do not stop to evaluate any change effort before 12 full weeks are over. At the end of 12 weeks, congratulate yourself on your achievement. If, at that point, you choose not to continue with the change or you slip back to old habits, you still will have increased your sense of self-respect, for in reaching this point you have succeeded in being true to your commitment. And you will have gained confidence in your ability to make other changes that may work better for you in the future.

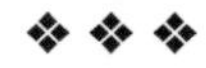

Experience the Transformation

Now it's time to put the rubber to the road. You've learned your health risks, you know the goals you want to reach, and you've made a plan you are willing to carry out for 12 full weeks. Let the games begin!

> *You do not have to be perfect to be successful in mastering behavioral change. Set your goals wisely and time will effect the changes without any further effort on your part other than a willingness to stay true to your plan. Once your plan is made, don't question what you are doing or reconsider what you have chosen. Be faithful to yourself.*

Give yourself 12 full weeks. You may feel the change has taken root at 10 weeks—great. Or you may not really feel solid in the change until week 14—

fine. *At whatever point the change happens for you, you will know it and from that point on, your behavior will be become much, much easier to maintain. It fact, your whole life will begin to get easier and easier—and more fun.* In choosing some smart goals and then sticking to behaviors that will achieve them, you will end up a happier and more powerful person—*guaranteed.*

Whenever the change happens for you, whether at week 10, 12, or 14, you will arrive at the threshold of a whole new set of possibilities. You will feel the power of your own ability to self-direct your destiny. You will discover that you can be exactly as you choose to be, in any aspect of your life.

So what's it like living through change during those first 12 weeks? If you approach your effort as the most important thing in your life—which it is—you will be very focused. If you have chosen your goals and behaviors wisely, you will feel both confident and a little nervous about your plan. You will know you can do it, but you will be nervous about failing. That nervousness is good. It will help keep you excited and dedicated to not deviating from your plan.

During your first four weeks, you will tend to your plan as if it were a small child that you are trying to protect. You will try hard to be perfect and not to waver at all from your goal. This is a good approach. Since you are trying to behave in new and different ways, you are learning each day to do new things or do old things differently. However, as with all learning, it takes practice and some extra time before the changes begin to feel natural and like second nature. Getting off to a good start in the first four weeks will help you as you get into the second four weeks.

During the second four weeks, you will see that the plan is starting to work, life is going on, and you are succeeding. Things are still a little new, and you may feel at times like abandoning your new behaviors for old, more comfortable patterns. It is at this juncture you must put all your trust in the simple passage of time. Whether you are loving what's happening or hating it, just keep doing it until your 12 weeks are completed. *Do not stop to re-evaluate at this point!* You might have a couple of lapses during this time, but don't feel that they are derailing you from your plan. Remember, perfection is not required! You still will achieve your goal even with a few lapses. Stay focused on finishing the 12 weeks.

The third and final four weeks are fun. You are definitely seeing and feeling changes in your life and how you feel. Things are getting easier and you do not have to pay such close attention. Things may not totally seem second nature yet, but they are starting to happen on their own. You may still have occasional urges to relapse to old behaviors, but your new behaviors are beginning to feel more comfortable, and you can live without constantly attending to them. In fact, your new behaviors are starting to feel preferable to your old ones, and you don't want to go back to the way you were doing things before. You are starting to realize that you can make any lifestyle change you choose because you are now skilled not only in the change you have just made, but in the whole behavioral change process.

Once you reduce a single health risk with a single lifestyle change that you are willing to sustain, you have all the skills you need to make any other behavior changes you choose. You can then start to think of your health risks like those little tin duck targets in shooting booths at county fairs. Up to this point, we have been concerned about 12 weeks as an initial phase of change. There are four 12-week cycles in a single year. If you have a lot of health risks and a number of behavior changes you would like to make, by using 12-week plans, the progress you can make in a single year can be amazing. Do one 12-week cycle first, and you will see just how true this is.

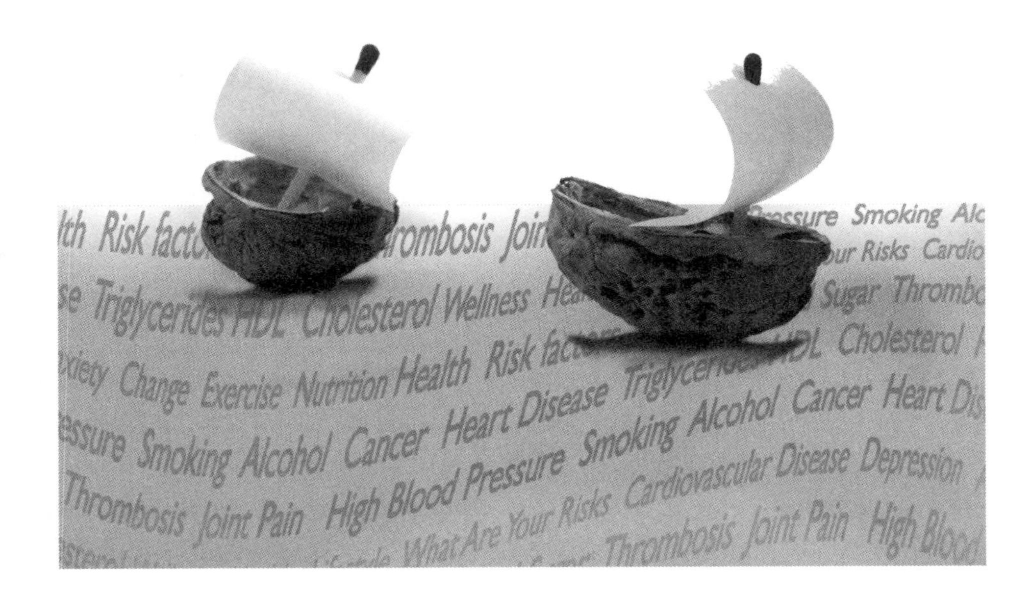

Good Health in a Nutshell

The following is an optimal health checklist for you to take to your health-care provider and use as a guide for determining your health risks, setting goals, and maintaining your health.

Blood Pressure (optimal)

- Systolic Blood Pressure (SBP)—Less than or equal to 120
- Diastolic Blood Pressure (DBP)—Less than 80

Cholesterol

- Total Cholesterol—Less than 200
- Triglycerides—Less than 150
- HDL (good cholesterol)—Men greater than 50, women greater than 55

- LDL (bad cholesterol)—At least below 130 and current thinking is the lower the better down to below 70
- VLDL (very low, very bad)—Less than 30

Weight

- Body Mass Index—less than or equal to 25
- Weight Loss—If a BMI of 25 is not a reasonable goal, losing 10 to 15 percent of your current body weight pays huge health benefits even if you remain overweight

Smoking

- Tobacco use—none in any form

Alcohol: use daily limits

- American Guideline—24 oz. beer, 10 oz. wine, 1 oz. hard liquor; ½ that for women
- UK Guideline—safe amount depends on age, size, sex, and health. Men should drink no more than 21 units of alcohol per week (and no more than four units in any one day). Women should drink no more than 14 units of alcohol per week (and no more than three units in any one day). Units: Strong beer at 6 percent abv (alcohol by volume) has six units in one liter. If you drink half a liter (500 ml)—just under a pint—then you have had three units. Wine at 12 percent abv has 12 units in one liter. If you drink a quarter of a liter (250 ml —two small glasses), then you have had three units.
- Consensus Guideline—drinking every day and drinking more than one or two drinks increases risk.

Anxiety and Stress

- Average score of 3 or less on the Stress / Anxiety scale

  In general, my stress / anxiety level is:

  1-very low
  2-somewhat low
  3-normal (neither high nor low)
  4-somewhat high
  5-high
  6-very high

Depression

- Average score of 3 or less on the Depression scale:
  For the last two weeks I have felt:
  1-not at all depressed
  2-not depressed
  3-neither depressed nor not depressed
  4-a little depressed
  5-more depressed than not depressed
  6-very depressed

Metabolic Syndrome

- Having three to five of the following risks: high triglycerides, low HDL, high blood pressure, insulin insensitivity, central obesity.
- Triglycerides less than 150 (with medication for those in the 300 to 1,000 range); HDL greater than 50 in men, 55 in women; BP less than 120 / 80 (average your monthly readings); fasting glucose less than 100; waist measurement less than 40 inches in men, less than 35 inches in women and waist / hip ratio greater than 0.9 in men and 0.8 in women (see weight loss goals on the previous page if waist measurement and waist / hip ratio is not a reasonable goal).

Diabetes

- Fasting Blood Sugar less than 100
- All Non-Fasting Blood Sugars between 80 and 160
- Hemoglobin A1c less than or equal to 6 to 6.5

Cancer

- Regular screenings to include PAP smears, mammograms, prostate exams, colonoscopy, skin surveys, plus regular healthcare and checkups are up to date even if you are well.
- Control weight, get adequate exercise, don't smoke, eat a healthy, low-fat diet with lots of whole foods—particularly fruits and vegetables in a variety of colors.

Exercise

- Walking, biking, swimming, and / or running at least 240 minutes per week (or more) performed at your target heart rate, plus stretching and weight work.

Nutrition

- A diet consisting mostly of whole, unprocessed foods that is low in fat, sugar, and sodium and high in fruits, vegetables, fiber, potassium, and water. Enjoy foods from all food groups, including carbohydrates, proteins, dairy products, fruits, vegetables, legumes, healthy fats, and plenty of water. Consume the number of calories that will promote weight loss, weight gain, or weight maintenance based on individual needs.

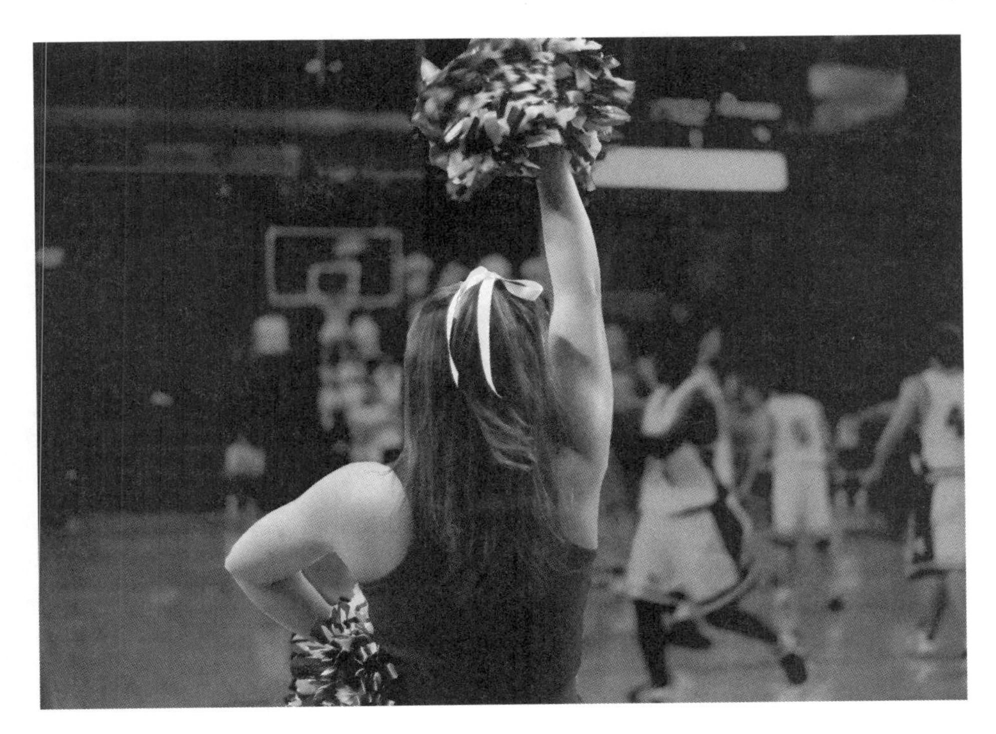

A Final Pep Talk

HEALTH RISKS ARE BEST MANAGED IN PARTNERSHIP with your healthcare provider. Health choices are those behaviors that you can employ in your everyday life that tip the risk balance away from illness toward a life of health and wellness.

By incorporating simple habits like taking your medications properly, getting more fresh air and exercise, and eating more fruits and vegetables, you can *significantly* improve your health. By taking on tougher challenges such as quitting smoking, losing weight, or conquering an addiction, you can unleash your personal power and discover your own inner strength. It is possible to change the entire direction of your life if that is what you want.

The journey to good health starts with a vision of your destination. Find a point in front of you to steer toward; create a picture in your mind of the kind of life you want to live. Once you go through the process of identifying your unique risk factors for disease, you will decide if you want to make changes in your life to reduce them.

> *You can achieve your goals. Believe you will fulfill your vision, and you will arrive at a point of satisfaction with your life because of your efforts.*

The thing about a journey from unhealthy to healthy living is that it doesn't have to feel like deprivation. You can still enjoy most of the things you do right now, but you will do so *in moderation*. You will limit, not banish, things like high-calorie, high-fat foods, and time in front of the TV or computer. You will balance less healthy habitual behaviors with opposing healthier habits like lower total calorie consumption, more time outdoors, more physical activity, and so on. In time, these new balancing behaviors will make you feel better, and you will not want to give them up. They will allow you to enjoy your favorite foods and activities in a balanced way without their causing you harm. By continually striving for this sense of balance, you can find pleasure and meaning in all your activities and behaviors. You will control your pleasures; they will not control you.

If you can grasp firmly the vital life force within you and use it to attack the unhealthy behaviors in your life, you will be shocked at your strength and abilities. And in starting with a clear picture of where you want to finish, you are already closer to success than you can imagine.

Healthy lives and healthy behaviors are circular.

As you replace old unhealthy behaviors with new healthier ones, the healthy ones tend to circle back on themselves to create more healthy behaviors. For example, if you are exercising regularly, you will tend to eat in a more healthy way that will help your exercise performance. If you are trying to quit smoking and don't want to gain weight, you will tend to exercise more to distract you from your cravings and prevent weight gain. If you are watching your sodium intake to control your blood pressure, you will be more likely to take your medications properly so you can achieve the blood pressure control you are seeking.

Unhealthy behaviors, too, circle back on themselves in the same way.

Let's say your goal is to lose weight and be more active. You have decided to achieve this by going for a walk each night after dinner. You have a long day at work and skip lunch. Because you're so hungry on your way home, you drive through for a super size meal at a fast food restaurant. You know this dinner won't help with your goal to lose weight, so now it's easy to abandon your exercise goal and skip the evening's walk. You completely cave in to your more familiar and comfortable sedentary life the moment you walk through the door, switching on the TV and popping a beer. You tell yourself, "Tomorrow I'll eat better and walk."

An additional problem with this scenario is that it is accompanied by a sense of failure, regret, and self-loathing. The unhealthy behaviors tend to perpetuate themselves, as does the negative self-talk that goes with not acting on the goals you have set for yourself. You tell yourself, "I'm weak, undisciplined; I have no will-power." And so, in addition to continuing unhealthy behaviors that cause physical illness, you are creating an inner life that puts you at risk for mental illness. Depression and anxiety find fertile ground in an atmosphere of such negative self-talk.

This brings us to an essential element of human life and, in fact, the very source of inner strength: the unseen world. It can also be thought of as the voice within or the inner monologue. As human beings we have the ability to reflect, imagine, and create images in our mind's eye.

Stop and think about how much time you spend in the unseen world of your imagination. While sitting in traffic, while waiting in lines, while drifting off to sleep at night, you are living in an unseen world. Miracles occur because of the imaginings of human minds.

Who can possibly say the unseen world is not real? There is evidence of it everywhere. From art to religion to physics to philosophy, the greatest achievements of the world were born first in human minds long before others saw them. Think of what Leonardo da Vinci saw in his unseen world. Think of what author J.K. Rowling saw in her unseen world in order to bring Harry Potter and his adventures to the rest of us. Think of how painters, sculptors, composers, writers, actors, architects, and designers see their creations in a world unseen by others before they bring their vision to reality. And think, too, about the joy that these artists and visionaries experience as they labor to create their unseen worlds for the rest of us to see.

It is in your unseen inner world that you invent yourself and create your life. How you perceive the world, what you imagine, what you think about make you who you are. You and I can both go into nature. What you see and feel there is beautiful. You can feel a spiritual presence infusing your soul, enriching and comforting you, and you have a deeply pleasurable experience. You do not sense what I sense. I see only a bunch of trees, and not the dappled sunlight through the leaves. I'm hot and don't feel a subtle breeze. My mind is on what traffic will be like driving back and what I want for dinner. While we are in the same place, looking at the same things, we are having totally different experiences.

What does this have to do with healthy living and behavior change?

> *Once you have identified your risks in order to make changes and reduce those risks, you will need to reinvent yourself. You will need to think differently about who you are and how you want to live.*

If your present lifestyle has created health risks such as increased weight or elevated blood pressure and you do not wish to change, those problems are likely to get worse. As those problems worsen, you are at increased risk for more serious problems, and so the circular process leading to more health problems continues until some catastrophic event happens. If that catastrophic event occurs, you will likely regret you didn't make efforts to prevent it sooner.

On the other hand, if you choose to see and imagine yourself healthy, and you undertake those behaviors that will promote your health, your unseen world becomes a more positive and inspiring place. It begins to support and nourish you; it gives you strength to do things you didn't think you could do.

Seemingly by magic, you begin to see changes in yourself and your world—both the seen and unseen parts. You start feeling better about yourself. You begin to feel in control of yourself and your life. You begin to imagine better things for yourself. You start to dream dreams and believe you can make them come true. Infused with this kind of strength, you recognize that reducing your risk factors for disease is just a first step.

Discovering your true, authentic self and manifesting that self in your world becomes your mission and your destiny. That is when you know you've reached the end, and that you have only just begun your journey.

Building a healthy life is like climbing a mountain. The challenge is always before you and there is effort involved. Look for things to hold on to, handholds and footholds that feel solid and that you trust. Once you've found them, climb steadily moving from one hold to the next, ever ascending, until at last you reach the summit—satisfaction with your health and comfort in your life.

Your health rests in your hands and in the hands of your Maker. There is much in life you cannot control. To handle the unexpected and prevail over adversity, you need faith and trust in your power to endure.

Faith comes from the heart. The power to endure comes from your ability to remain agile and to adapt to changing circumstances. Change happens; it can't be stopped. The passage of time cannot be slowed or halted. We all grow old (if we are lucky). How well you age is largely up to you. It is the intention of this book to give you all the knowledge and tools you need so you can age to perfection.

There are things you can control and things you can't. This book has tried to guide you down a clear path that will maximize health and happiness throughout your life. It is my hope that you may have a life that begins with a happy childhood, grows into a vigorous and productive adulthood, and concludes in a peaceful and wise old age. The belief that this is possible motivated the writing of this book.

Those whose lives are happiest continue to grow and change until the end. A capacity for change, plus good humor and a sense of optimism, can lift even the heaviest burden and bring comfort through the darkest of nights.

Whether you have worked through this book sequentially or reviewed only those chapters of interest, I hope you have learned something about your health, your health risks, and the healthcare you need. You now have the information you need to make choices about how you can improve your health today and reduce your risk of disease in the future.

There is no one right way for everyone.

It's a puzzle figuring out what path to health and happiness is the right one. You now possess important knowledge that will help you determine the right way for you. Whatever your size, shape, age, or risk profile, there is a life you are meant to live. Don't miss your chance to live it by anesthetizing yourself with addictions or unhealthy behaviors.

> *Life is fleeting. Every sunrise and sunset is unique. Every day that you are without illness, addiction, and debility is a day to treasure and be grateful for.*

Those days that are clouded by adversity, pain, and grief have their lessons, too. At the end of long periods of trouble and darkness, peace and light can follow. Don't dull your experiences with denial or addiction. Relish the joy. Admire the good. Endure the pain. Accept the fear. Feel the grief. And know that all—both darkness and light—will be part of your life.

Have the courage to make up your own mind about things. Don't buy everything you are sold. Don't measure yourself by the things you own or the money you make. Don't think that food or drink or drugs or money or makeovers or sex are going to make you happy. It's inner peace; it's being playful; it's loving people and having them love you back; it's breathing clean air; it's moving your body through space; it's laughter; it's generosity; it's integrity; it's honesty; it's kindness; it's self-respect; it's fighting for a greater good—these are things that will make you happy. They'll keep you healthy, too.

> *Good luck on your journey. Remember, everything is possible. Live long with good health.*

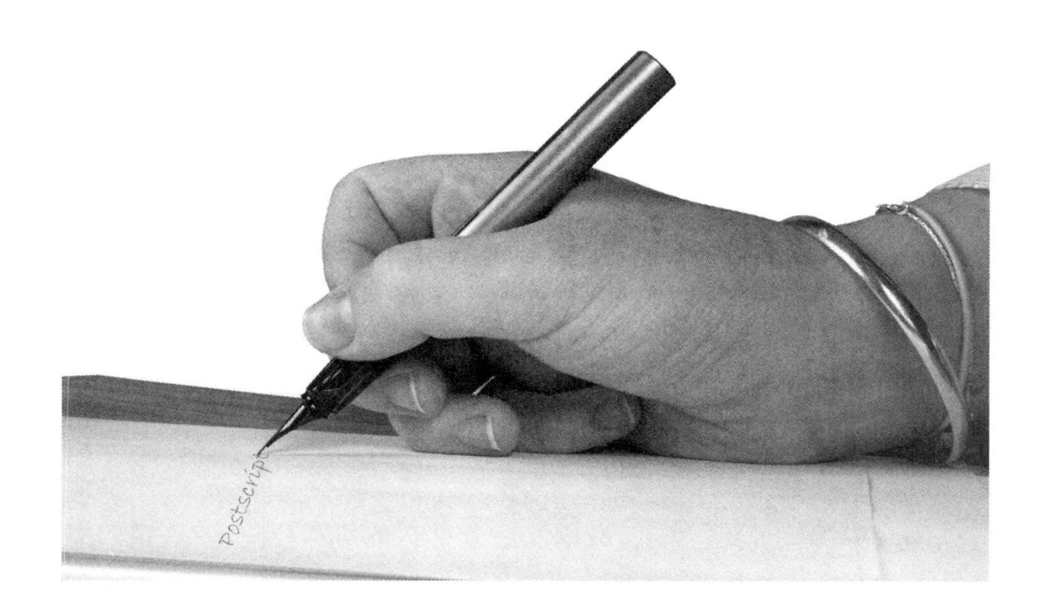

Postscript

Here are the facts. Five preventable diseases cause two-thirds of the deaths in the United States. A staggering 75 percent of the nation's total healthcare cost is spent treating heart attacks and strokes, diabetes, chronic lung disease, and cancer. Imagine the savings in human suffering and dollars if these diseases were controlled or prevented.

According to the American Journal of Health Promotion, only one out of five American adults today has good mental and physical health. The other four out of five are getting sick and / or dying from preventable diseases. Sadly, that means more than 65 percent of Americans will die needlessly from diseases they could prevent themselves. Unfortunately, most people do not know how to take the simple, personal life-saving steps to reduce their risk factors for serious disease. But with proper guidance and adequate self-care, it is possible to avoid or at least control most of these diseases. By learning about them, it is possible not only to achieve better health, but also to receive better healthcare.

The hard truth is that most of the more than 80 million aging baby boomers in this country are not aging well. Obesity is an epidemic. Diabetes is on the rise at alarming rates. Our social norms promote high-fat, fast-food diets, and sedentary lifestyles. Until the healthcare system in America turns its attention to disease prevention and health promotion, until we consumers stop buying from (and thus enriching) companies whose products sicken and kill us, health in America will continue to decline. And, until individuals and groups make a conscious and informed effort toward risk factor reduction, we, as a people, will continue to get sicker and sicker at higher and higher costs.

There is a better way. We can start making smarter health choices.

You can get started by reading this book and then taking what you have learned from it to heart. Those mavericks among us who choose to buck the current norms and forge healthy lifestyles for ourselves will have the best chance to prosper and thrive.

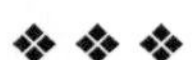

Maverick Health was founded to offer care to everyone who chooses to live better, hopes to live longer, and wishes to do so with good health. Contact us at:

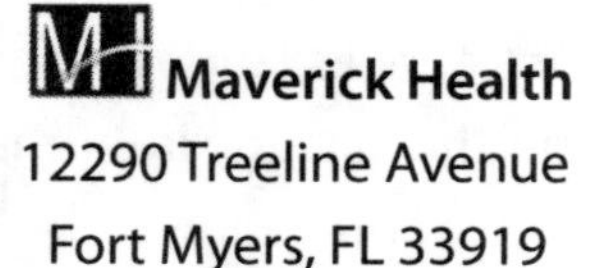

12290 Treeline Avenue
Fort Myers, FL 33919
Phone: (800) 595-2315
email: info@MaverickHealth.com
website: www.MaverickHealth.com

Appendix

Reference of Health Risks

Take what you can use
and let the rest go by.

— *Ken Kesey*

Appendix

Contents

Routine Laboratory Tests

The following information is provided to explain in simple terms the general purpose and normal values for routine blood and urine tests. It is by no means a complete list of all the laboratory and diagnostic tests used to establish medical diagnoses. To find out the specific tests for specific health risks, see the corresponding sections outlined in later pages in this Appendix.

Different laboratories use slightly different ranges for "normal," called *reference ranges*. This means that the ranges you see on your test reports might vary a little from those listed here. The reference ranges used here are from the *Textbook of Primary Care Medicine, 2nd edition* (Editor-in-Chief, John Noble, M.D.; Mosby, Inc., 1996). Small variations, either above or below the normal ranges listed here, may or may not be important in your case. This information is *not* intended to replace the advice of your healthcare provider, nor does it completely cover all the implications of the tests described. Discuss any abnormal lab values and their significance with your provider.

Tests are ways to measure, obtain images of, and assess various substances and structures in your body. They include everything from simple blood and urine tests and x-rays, to sophisticated tests like CT (computed tomography) scans, MRI (magnetic resonance imaging) scans, biopsies, and others. The chart that follows lists the routine blood and urine tests with the reference (normal) ranges for them. You can compare your own tests against this chart to see if yours seem normal. However, you should see your health provider to get an explanation of any abnormal results and to get advice on whether or not they need treatment.

As mentioned earlier, there are hundreds of tests not included here. Some of the more specialized tests are discussed in the sections that deal with the diseases for which these tests are used.

Routine lab tests reveal a lot about how your body is functioning and whether there are abnormalities that require further investigation. Try to keep a file at home with copies of all your lab tests. Your healthcare provider should be happy to give you copies. If you keep your own file, you will always have your test results available if you move or see a new provider.

Laboratory tests are only one part of your assessment. They are most useful when evaluated in light of your medical history, physical examination, vital signs, and current health status along with any symptoms you are having.

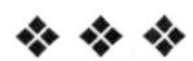

Your Routine Blood and Urine Tests

CBC (Complete Blood Cell) Count

There are two main kinds of blood cells: red and white. Red blood cells carry oxygen; white blood cells fight infections.

The CBC consists of a series of tests on a single specimen of your blood and measures the following:

- The *total number* of blood cells (how many red cells and how many white cells) per cubic milliliter of whole blood
- The *size* of the blood cells
- The *percentage* of different specialized types of blood cells in the total number of cells
- The *concentration* of blood cells in the plasma. (Think of separate particles, some shaped like tiny balls and some shaped like lozenges, all floating around in water. The particles are the blood cells and the water is plasma. The concentration is how many of the particles there are in a certain volume of water. More particles mean higher concentration; fewer particles mean lower concentration.)

The CBC is a common screening and diagnostic blood test. It is used to diagnose conditions such as anemia, viral or bacterial infections, immune system abnormalities, and other disorders that affect your blood. It is a useful test that can monitor your response to treatments and track the course of certain illnesses.

CBC Values

Total white blood cell (WBC) count	4.5 to 11 (cells x 10^9 / L)
Total erythrocyte (red blood cell) count	4.6 to 6.2 (cells x 10^{12} / L)
Hemoglobin (lower in women, higher in men)	12 to 18 g / dl
Hematocrit (lower in women, higher in men)	38% to 52%
MCV (mean corpuscular volume)	82 to 98 (fL)
MCH (mean corpuscular hemoglobin)	27 to 32 (pg)
MCHC (mean corpuscular hemoglobin concentration)	32 to 36 g / dl
Reticulocyte count (immature blood cells)	0.5% to 2.5% of erythrocyte total
Platelet count (important for blood clotting)	150 to 350 (cells x 10^9 / L)

WBC Differential Values
(WBC subtypes as a percentage of the total WBC count)

Segmented neutrophils	40% to 60%
Banded neutrophils	0% to 3%
Eosinophils	0% to 5%
Basophils	0% to 1%
Lymphocytes	20% to 45%
Monocytes	2% to 6%

Electrolytes

These are also called "lytes." They are important chemicals in your body. Electrolytes are present both in your bloodstream (*extra*cellular) and inside the cells of your body (*intra*cellular). These chemical particles move back and forth, in and out, from your blood to your cells, and from your cells to your blood. They keep the balance of fluids in your body constant and stable. They keep the chemistry of your body regulated. They allow your body to function properly.

A healthy body regulates electrolytes automatically. Certain conditions, such as kidney problems, excessive diarrhea or vomiting, hormonal abnormalities, and medication side effects, can alter the electrolyte balance in your body. If electrolyte abnormalities become severe enough, they can even cause death. The following are the main electrolytes.

<table>
<tr>
<td>Potassium is present in small amounts in your blood, but in large amounts inside your cells (because it is intracellular). It has the following important functions:
• It influences the excitability of your nerves and muscles.
• It regulates water inside the cells of your body.
• It affects tissue growth and repair.
• It maintains your body's proper acid-base chemistry.
If your potassium is too low, it is called hypokalemia. This can cause muscle weakness, even paralysis, and can stop your heart from beating. If your potassium is too high, it is called hyperkalemia. This can cause abnormal heart rhythms or stop your heart from beating. Both conditions are very dangerous and can be life-threatening.</td>
<td>3.5 to
5.2 mEq / L</td>
</tr>
</table>

Sodium is present in large amounts in your blood, but in small amounts in your cells (because it is *extracellular*). The main thing sodium does in your body is to maintain fluid balance. You can think of water being drawn to sodium particles. If you have a lot of sodium in your blood, you will have more water (or plasma), too. That is why a diet high in sodium (salt) tends to cause conditions like high blood pressure (because of higher blood volume), swelling in the legs, and generalized fluid retention. In a healthy person on a normal diet, the amount of sodium ingested is matched by the amount of sodium lost from the body, and sodium balance is maintained. Hyponatremia, or low sodium, is usually the result of drinking too much water or a hormonal abnormality. Hypernatremia, or high sodium, is usually the result of not drinking enough water or a hormonal abnormality. The kidneys are vital organs that regulate sodium. Kidney disease will also cause sodium abnormalities.	135 to 145 mEq / L
Chloride works along with sodium to regulate the fluid balance in your body. *Sodium chloride* is a chemical combination of both. The table salt we put on our food is sodium chloride.	95 to 105 mEq / L
Carbon dioxide (CO_2) is the fourth value reported in an electrolyte blood panel. Its main function is to regulate the acid-base balance in your body. The chemistry behind this is very complicated and beyond the scope of this book.	18 to 30 mmol / L

For our purposes here, it is important to know that electrolyte values are usually normal in a healthy person. If yours are abnormal, they can give your healthcare provider important clues as to the cause of your illness.

Routine Chemistry

Test	Normal range
Glucose is a type of sugar. A glucose test checks for diabetes, among other conditions. You should be *fasting* for this test. That means you have nothing to eat or drink (except water) after dinner on the night before your blood is drawn.	Fasting = 70 to 100 mg / dl Non-Fasting = 60 to 180 mg / dl
BUN (blood urea nitrogen) tests your kidney function. If it is high, you may be dehydrated or have eaten too much protein. If it is low, it may be from drinking too much water or other causes.	5 to 22 mg / dl
Creatinine also tests your kidney function. It is a critical lab test in the evaluation of renal (kidney) failure.	0.5 to 1.3 mg / dl
Calcium in your *blood* is an electrolyte that is involved with muscle and heart activity and the transmission of nerve signals. Certain hormonal conditions and diseases can cause abnormal blood levels of calcium. (Note: Most of the calcium in your body is found in your bones and teeth; calcium stored in the bones is not considered an electrolyte and cannot be measured with a blood test.)	8.7 to 10.6 mg / dl
Magnesium is found mostly in your bones, as well as inside your cells. Like calcium, it is an electrolyte that is involved with nerve and muscular activity. In addition, it plays a role in blood clotting and is also part of various enzyme systems. (An enzyme is a protein inside the cells of your body that causes chemical reactions to occur.) Magnesium is also involved with the metabolism of sugars and the production of proteins and other substances in your body. Magnesium and calcium are closely related and interact with each other.	1.5 to 2.5 mEq / L

In this table, < means less than, and > means greater than.

Phosphorus is an electrolyte that is closely related to calcium in your body. It, too, can be altered by both kidney disease and hormonal conditions.	2.0 to 4.3 mg / dl
Alk Phos (alkaline phosphatase) is an enzyme. A high alk phos level can indicate liver or bone disease when it is related to other abnormalities. Alk phos can also become high from medications and other conditions. It is *always* high in young, growing children and pregnant women, and does not represent illness in those cases.	35 to 125 IU / L
LDH (lactic acid dehydrogenase) is another enzyme found all over your body. The LDH test is not a specific test. That means that several things can cause high LDH levels. Leakage of LDH into your bloodstream results in increased levels. LDH is one marker (although not the most specific) for a heart attack. Weight lifting can increase your level a lot. This is because lifting weights tears your skeletal muscles, and when you have torn muscles, LDH is released from your muscles into your bloodstream.	20 to 220 IU / L
CK (creatine kinase) is an enzyme very similar to LDH (above). It also is not a specific test. A special CK test called a *CK-MB* test is a very specific marker for cardiac muscle damage and is used when diagnosing and treating a heart attack. A plain CK test can be elevated by weight lifting (as with LDH, above) because of its presence in skeletal muscle. This test is also used to check for muscle damage that can be caused by some medications, like statins. (See the High Cholesterol section in this Appendix.)	20 to 200 IU / L

Total protein is a measurement of all the different types of proteins found in your blood. You get proteins through your diet, then your body breaks them down and reassembles them into many different types of proteins that have many different functions. Proteins are needed for tissue repair and immune system functions, and they function as "carriers" that transport other substances around your body. Total protein is a good test to assess your general health. It is also an indicator of a number of different diseases including kidney and liver problems, abnormal functioning of your immune system, inflammatory conditions, and malnutrition.	6.0 to 8.3 g / dl
Albumin is one type of protein in your body. It is called a *serum protein* because it is mostly found in your bloodstream. One of its main purposes is to maintain your blood volume. Remember, we talked about sodium pulling water (or plasma) into your bloodstream; well, albumin does this much more powerfully. Very low levels of albumin will result in swelling, usually of your lower legs, called *edema*. This results from water leaking out of your bloodstream and into soft tissues because there is not enough albumin in your blood vessels to keep the fluid there. The scientific name for this is *oncotic pressure*. Albumin is also an important transport protein, helping substances dissolve in your blood by binding to them so they can move around your body.	3.0 to 5.5 g / dl

Globulin is another type of protein. There are five types of globulins, and they have many functions. HDL cholesterol and LDL cholesterol (described under Cholesterol Profile) are globulins called lipoproteins. Globulins bind to other chemicals to transport them through your body and are also involved in blood cell production and clotting. Finally, globulins make up the immunoglobulins that defend our bodies against foreign substances and disease-causing organisms.	2.4 to 3.5 g / dl
SGOT / AST (aspartate aminotransferase) is a liver function test. Usually the ALT and AST are done together. The AST is more sensitive for detecting cell damage and increases more than the ALT if you have acute hepatitis or alcoholism. Because AST is also present in heart muscle, it will increase after a heart attack, too.	5 to 40 U / L
SGPT / ALT (alanine aminotransferase) is a liver function test. It is an enzyme that, when high, indicates damage to your liver. It is used to diagnose and monitor liver diseases such as hepatitis and cirrhosis. This test will be done if you start taking certain medications, like the statins used to treat high cholesterol. Most medications are metabolized by your liver, and it is important to know your liver is healthy and functioning properly before you start taking certain ones. Chronic alcohol abuse can increase your ALT, too.	0 to 40 U / L

Bilirubin is a by-product of the breakdown of the hemoglobin in your red blood cells. Our bodies are constantly breaking down old cells and making new ones. Bilirubin is removed from your body by your liver, which excretes it into your bile. Increased levels may indicate liver disease or a blockage. If your levels are high, you may get yellowing of your skin and the whites of your eyes, called *jaundice*.	0.2 to 1.2 mg / dl
Uric acid is a waste product. It comes from the breakdown of proteins in your body called *purines*. Your kidneys normally excrete two-thirds of it; one-third is excreted in your stool. A high uric acid level may indicate that your body can't excrete it, signaling kidney disease. Another cause of increased uric acid levels is gout. High levels can be caused by other diseases, too, such as increased destruction of your cells from starvation, dieting, or leukemia.	2.0 to 9.0 mg / dl
Homocysteine is an amino acid (a chemical building block of proteins) that is a by-product of normal protein breakdown. High levels of homocysteine are believed to increase your risk of coronary artery disease; the levels can be lowered by treatment with high doses of folic acid and B vitamins.	5.0 to 12 μmol / L
C-reactive protein (CRP) is a plasma protein that rises in response to inflammation. Increased levels are believed to increase your risk of cardiovascular disease. If your levels are high, taking 81 mg of aspirin daily (if you are not allergic or have other reasons you should not take aspirin) may reduce risk.	<0.6 mg / L

<table>
<tr>
<td>TSH (thyroid-stimulating hormone) is a hormone that is made by your pituitary gland in your brain. It regulates the production of thyroid hormone by your thyroid gland; that hormone, in turn, influences your metabolism. TSH works on what is called a negative feedback system.

If your body is not making enough thyroid hormone (you have a low level), your TSH goes up. This in effect tells your thyroid gland to "make more hormone." So a high TSH means you have a low thyroid hormone level (hypothyroidism). If you are hypothyroid, you may feel sluggish, be constipated, gain weight, have no energy, and be depressed.

If your TSH is low, that is because it is suppressed by too much thyroid hormone in your body (hyperthyroidism). If you are hyperthyroid, you may feel anxious, have trouble sleeping, have diarrhea, and lose weight.

Thyroid function is routinely checked with a TSH test. If your thyroid function is abnormal, there are treatments that can help regulate it.</td>
<td>0.2 to 5.4 microunits/ml (IU/L SI units)</td>
</tr>
<tr>
<td>Hemoglobin A1c is a component of red blood cells that carries sugar in the blood. It is used to measure an average blood sugar over the previous three months to evaluate blood sugar control in people with diabetes.</td>
<td>Non-Diabetic:
4.0 to 5.9%
Diabetic Goal:
<6.0 to 6.5%</td>
</tr>
</table>

Cholesterol Profile

Note: This test is discussed in detail in the High Cholesterol section in this Appendix. There is also more about cholesterol on page 55. The important thing to know here is that your blood should be drawn first thing in the morning when you have had nothing to eat or drink—except water or black coffee—after dinner the night before. The following are explanations of the four parts of the cholesterol profile.

Total cholesterol is a measure of all the types of cholesterol in your body.	< 200 mg / dl
Triglycerides are fats circulating in your blood. This measurement is variable; it can be "high" after a high-fat meal and "normal" after a fast. Triglycerides cannot be measured accurately unless you are fasting.	< 150 mg / dl
HDL (high-density lipoprotein) cholesterol is the "good" cholesterol. This cholesterol actually protects you from the hazards of high cholesterol. Because of its high density, HDL rolls through your blood vessels like a bowling ball, knocking off plaque and helping keep your arteries clean. The higher your HDL is, the better.	> 40 mg / dl in men > 50 mg / dl in women
LDL (low-density lipoprotein) cholesterol is the "bad" cholesterol. This is the gooey stuff, like sludge, that sticks to the walls of your arteries and buries itself inside them, clogging them up. The normal LDL value depends on your other risk factors, but the lower the better.	< 70 to 100 mg / dl (See the High Cholesterol section.)

In this table, < means less than, and > means greater than.

Routine Urinalysis

This is a very useful test that can detect abnormalities requiring further follow-up. The routine urinalysis tests the properties of your urine, particularly its color, clarity, concentration, and acidity. In addition, it tests for substances that should not be present in normal urine. Your urine is examined with the naked eye, under a microscope, and with chemical reagent strips that, when dipped in urine, detect the presence of specific chemicals.

How to obtain a "clean catch" specimen: Using the clean catch method is important for collecting urine without contaminating it with bacteria. First, wash your hands. Next, clean your genital area well with towelettes that should be provided. The urethral opening is where the urine comes out. It should be cleaned of all bacteria that may be on the outside of your skin before giving the specimen. Do *not* touch the inside of the specimen container. If you have to set the cap down, make sure that it is facing *up* so as not to contaminate the inside of the top of the specimen container.

Color should be pale yellow to amber. Urine that is red or dark brown is abnormal. The darkness of the color tells how well hydrated you are. If you are dehydrated, it will be very dark. If you are well hydrated, it will be lighter.	Yellow (versus brown or red)
Appearance measures the clarity of your urine. It should be clear. Cloudy urine, particularly if it also has a foul odor, may signal bacteria in your urine and a urinary infection.	Clear (versus cloudy)
Specific gravity measures the concentration of your urine and reflects how well hydrated you are. Values range from 1.003 (dilute) to 1.030 (concentrated). You can dilute your urine by drinking more water.	1.003 to 1.030
pH measures the acidity of your urine. It is normally slightly acidic (pH numbers below 7 are acidic; pH numbers above 7 are basic).	4.6 to 8.0

Protein is an abnormal finding. Your urine should not have any protein in it. Its presence may indicate kidney disease. People with high blood pressure sometimes have protein in their urine because of the high pressure under which their blood is pumped through their kidneys. There are other causes of protein in the urine, too. So its presence should always be followed up with your healthcare provider.	Negative
Urine glucose (sugar) is an abnormal finding. It usually indicates that you have diabetes. But urine glucose is a much less sensitive measure of diabetes than blood glucose (blood sugar); by the time glucose is getting into your urine, your blood sugar is *way* too high. That's why diabetes is now monitored by blood sugars and not urine sugars.	Negative
Ketones are an abnormal finding. They are the waste products of the metabolism of fats. In healthy people, ketones are formed in the liver and completely metabolized there, so they are absent from the urine. Ketones are found in the urine in people who have diabetes that is out of control, and this can be an early warning of a life-threatening complication called ketoacidosis, which can lead to coma and death in diabetics. Ketones are also found in the urine in people who eat high-fat, high-protein diets.	Negative
Urine bilirubin is an abnormal finding. Like ketones, this substance is usually completely metabolized in your liver. Its presence in your urine (and blood) may indicate liver disease (such as hepatitis and cirrhosis) or a blockage of the ducts from your gallbladder. Very high levels of bilirubin in your body result in a yellowing of your skin and the whites of your eyes, called jaundice.	Negative

Urobilinogen is a substance that comes from the breakdown of bilirubin. You should have only a tiny amount in your urine. A high level in your urine is one of the most sensitive indicators of abnormal liver function. Unlike bilirubin, urobilinogen is colorless and so will not cause jaundice.	0.0 to 0.2 EU / dl
Blood should not be present in your urine. The most common reasons for blood in your urine are a urinary tract infection (UTI), kidney stones, or menstruation in women. There can be other causes, too, such as slight trauma in men. If you have blood in your urine, you should keep having a urinalysis until your urine is free from blood. If the blood persists, you should be referred to a urologist.	Negative
Nitrites are by-products of bacteria. Their presence in your urine indicates a bacterial infection. Sometimes people have urinary tract infections without any symptoms. If your urine is positive for nitrites, you should have a urine culture and sensitivity test and be treated for an infection. You may still have an infection without nitrites in your urine, but positive nitrites means you have a urinary tract infection.	Negative
WBCs (white blood cells) may also indicate an infection. The presence of 50 or more white blood cells per high-powered field (HPF) under the microscope indicates infection. You may or may not have symptoms (like burning when you urinate, frequency, urgency, or feeling like your bladder is never emptied). If you have more than 50 WBCs in your urine, you should have a urine culture and sensitivity test. Discuss with your healthcare provider whether you should have treatment.	0 to 5 / HPF

RBCs (red blood cells) are sometimes found in the urine and may or may not indicate a problem. As noted under Blood, their presence may be caused by menstruation in women or slight trauma in men. If you have RBCs in your urine, you should keep having a urinalysis until your urine is clear of red blood cells.	0 to 5 / HPF
Squamous epithelial cells are cells that have sloughed off your body at the time the specimen was obtained. They indicate contamination of the urine specimen. A urinalysis that is positive for bacteria and WBCs, and has more than 50 squamous epithelial cells means the specimen is contaminated and you should collect a new specimen, using the "clean catch" method described earlier.	0 to 50 / HPF
Microalbumin measures the presence of protein in your urine with much greater sensitivity than a regular urine protein test. By the time protein shows up in a regular urine test, your protein level is way too high. The test for microalbumin detects the problem much, much earlier. A high level of microalbumin in your urine can indicate kidney disease from diabetes or uncontrolled high blood pressure. (See the High Blood Pressure and Diabetes sections in this Appendix for more.)	< 30 mg / day

The Health Risks

Heart Attack and Stroke

Heart Attack

A heart attack is also called a *coronary*, a *myocardial infarction,* or an *MI*. It is a blockage of one or more of your coronary arteries. These are the arteries that carry blood to your heart muscle.

A heart attack is caused by one of three events:

- A spasm (or constriction) of one or more of your coronary arteries.
- A gradual blockage of one or more arteries from the buildup of fat and cholesterol.
- A sudden blockage of one or more of the arteries because a piece of plaque broke off from the artery wall and lodged there.

Symptoms of Heart Attack

The following are the typical symptoms of a heart attack.

- Chest pain (it may be gripping, or feel like pressure or a dull ache). It may radiate (travel) to your neck, shoulders, or left or both arms. People sometimes describe chest pain from a heart attack as feeling like an "elephant sitting on my chest." Some people don't recognize chest pressure as pain and so ignore it. That is very dangerous.
- Shortness of breath or difficulty taking a deep breath.
- Abdominal pain that is often described as "heartburn."
- Nausea, sometimes with vomiting, sometimes not.
- Sweating that is not associated with heat or exertion. Feeling cold and clammy while at rest or with only slight exertion is a symptom of heart attack, particularly if you also have any chest discomfort.
- Dizziness.
- Blackouts or fainting.
- Fatigue.
- A pounding heart or a feeling of change in your heart rhythm.
- Feelings of panic or anxiety.
- Just a feeling of indigestion or "heartburn" with no other symptoms.

But sometimes *there are no symptoms at all.* This is called a *silent* heart attack. In addition, people often ignore or deny the symptoms of heart attack. This is very dangerous and results in many unnecessary deaths.

Women's Symptoms of Heart Attack

The symptoms of a heart attack may be somewhat different in women.

- A general malaise.
- Stomach upset or indigestion that is not relieved by vomiting.
- Back or abdominal pain.
- Flu-like symptoms.
- Shortness of breath.
- Dizziness.
- Fatigue.
- An odd or "not right" feeling.

Women may also *have no symptoms at all*, a silent heart attack.

Treatments for Heart Attack

Modern treatments for heart attack are time driven and depend on getting the blocked artery or arteries open *as soon as possible* to prevent heart muscle from dying. This is achieved in one of two ways.

One way is with a procedure called *direct angioplasty*, in which a wire is run through your groin directly to the blocked artery to open it up and restore blood flow. This procedure is described in the CVD section that follows.

The other way is by using powerful drugs often called *"clot-busting" drugs*, which help break up and dissolve the clot that is causing the blockage.

Which method is used in your case will depend on the capabilities of the hospital in which you are treated and the judgment of the cardiologist treating you.

Your cardiologist will probably also give you some or all of the treatments listed below.

- **Aspirin:** This medication is given because it helps thin your blood, which can help dissolve the clot. A dose of 325 mg chewed at the onset of symptoms can be lifesaving.
- **Oxygen:** This medication is given through a thin plastic tube placed in your nose or through a mask placed over your nose and mouth.

During a heart attack, your heart muscle is dying from lack of oxygen. Breathing more oxygen increases the amount of oxygen in your blood, which helps your heart. Note: If you are having a heart attack, lie very still and do not walk around when you feel chest pain, because moving around uses up more of the oxygen in your blood, so there is less for your heart.

- **Nitroglycerin ("nitro"):** This medication is a coronary artery vasodilator. That means it relaxes coronary arteries that are in spasm and makes constricted (narrow) vessels wider. As a result, there is increased blood flow and oxygen to your heart muscle. Nitroglycerin often relieves chest pain. Special Note: If you take Viagra (generic name: sildenafil), Levitra (vardenafil), Cialis (tadalafil), or other medications for erectile dysfunction, you *must not* take nitroglycerin medications (including nitro for chest pain, nitro patches, or nitro creams) or the medications Isordil and Imdur (generic name: isosorbide) *for at least 48 hours*. If you have taken Viagra, Cialis, or Levitra within 48 hours and then take nitroglycerin, there is a risk of severe low blood pressure and cardiovascular collapse that can lead to death. Notify emergency medical personal immediately if you have used these drugs in the past 48 hours.
- **Metoprolol:** This is a blood pressure medication. The brand name is Lopressor. It comes from a class of drugs called *beta-blockers*. (For more, see the High Blood Pressure section in this Appendix.) This medication decreases how hard your heart works and slows down your heart rate, so that your heart needs less oxygen.
- **Heparin:** This powerful blood thinner is given through an intravenous line (IV) to break up the clot and help the blood flow more easily. There are other clot-busting drugs that are used at the hospital to help stop a heart attack, too, such as Streptase, Activase, and Retavase. If you suffer a heart attack, whether you are treated with clot-busters or are taken for emergency cardiac catheterization will depend on the judgment of the cardiologist treating you and the capabilities of the hospital where you are treated.

Stroke

A stroke is also called a *brain attack, cerebrovascular accident*, or *CVA*. In a stroke, blood stops flowing to a part of your brain.

A stroke is caused by one of two events:

- *Blockage*, when a plaque breaks off and lodges in one of the small vessels of your brain. The plaque is from atherosclerosis.
- *Bleeding*, when a small vessel ruptures (usually because of long-standing or sudden high blood pressure). The bleeding vessel stops blood from reaching a certain part of your brain.

Symptoms of a Stroke

A stroke can cause many different symptoms, depending on how bad it is and which part of your brain is affected.

- Sudden onset of weakness or numbness of your face, arm, or leg (usually on just one side of your body).
- Sudden dimness of vision, double vision, or vision loss (especially in one eye).
- Sudden confusion.
- Sudden difficulty speaking or understanding speech.
- Sudden severe headache without an obvious cause.
- Sudden dizziness, unsteadiness, balance problems, or falls without an obvious cause.
- Collapse or loss of consciousness.

Medications for a Stroke

If your stroke is caused by a blood clot, the same powerful clot-busting drugs used for heart attacks can prevent permanent disability from stroke. But if your stroke is caused by bleeding, clot-busting drugs will make it worse. For this reason, you need a CT scan *before you can begin treatment*. That why it is so important that you go to the hospital as soon as your symptoms start. Certain treatments can make the stroke milder and even save your life, but they only work if you have them *within three hours* of the time when your symptoms start.

Cardiovascular Disease

Targets

Tests / Measurements	Target Number
Blood pressure	< 140 / 80 mm Hg
Cholesterol	< 200 mg / dl
Triglycerides	< 150 mg / dl
HDL cholesterol	> 50 mg / dl
LDL cholesterol	<100 mg / dl
Body Mass Index (BMI)	< or = 25
Tobacco use	None
Fasting blood sugar	< 100 mg / dl
Hemoglobin A1c (HbA1c)	< or = 6% – 6.5%
Male waist circumference	< 40 inches
Female waist circumference	< 35 inches
Exercise	> 240 min / week
Homocysteine	< 10 mmol / L
C-reactive protein (CRP)	< 1.0 mg / L

In this table < means less than and > means greater than.

The best way to slow or reverse cardiovascular disease is to reduce your risk factors by *getting your numbers to target*. You can assess your risk factors using this book and discussing your risks during a medical checkup by your healthcare provider.

Evaluation by your provider will include a history, a physical examination, and tests to obtain values for the target numbers. The following tests are recommended to determine if you are at risk for or already have cardiovascular disease.

Routine Screening Tests

- Fasting blood sugar
- CBC (complete blood cell) count
- Electrolytes
- Complete metabolic profile (including a thyroid profile, and liver and kidney function tests)

- Total cholesterol profile, and possibly an advanced lipoprotein panel
- Urinalysis

Cardiovascular Tests

- **A 12-lead electrocardiogram (an EKG or ECG):** This test checks for irregular heart rate, irregular heart rhythm, and problems with blood flow to your heart. It is a simple test performed in your healthcare provider's office while you lie quietly on an examination table. Sticky electrodes are placed on your chest, arms, and legs, and a machine prints a graph of your heart activity. It is painless. It is *not* a good test for detecting coronary artery disease or injury; for that, you need a stress test (described below).
- **Cardiac stress test:** This test should be performed if you:
    - Are male and over 45
    - Are female and over 55
    - Have ever had chest pain
    - Are a smoker
    - Have high blood pressure
    - Have high cholesterol
    - Have diabetes
    - Want to begin a vigorous exercise program

  A cardiologist (heart specialist) performs this special electrocardiogram (ECG). It is done while you are either walking on a treadmill (if you are physically able) or lying on a table receiving special drugs in your veins (if you are unable to walk on the treadmill). This test checks your heart while it is being stressed to see if you have hidden coronary artery disease. This is a better test than a regular ECG for discovering if you have coronary artery disease, but it is not perfect.
- **Carotid ultrasound:** This test should be done if your healthcare provider hears *bruits* (swishing sounds) in your neck with a stethoscope. It should also be performed regularly if you have other risks like high blood pressure, high cholesterol, diabetes, or other forms of cardiovascular disease. This test checks for narrowing of your carotid arteries. These are the large arteries in your neck that carry blood to your brain. For this test, gel is applied to your neck and a

metal ball is rolled over it. The ultrasound machine makes a picture showing the blood flow through your carotid arteries and can detect blockages. This test doesn't hurt.

- **Ankle / arm index:** This is a fancy way to measure your blood pressure. It measures differences in blood pressures in your arms and legs. This test detects decreased blood flow and peripheral vascular disease (narrowing of the smaller arteries in your arms and legs). It feels the same as having your blood pressure taken, but it is done on both arms and both legs. A computer calculates from the measurements whether the blood flow to your extremities is normal or decreased.
- **Echocardiography:** This test is also an ultrasound test and checks the pumping ability and shape of your heart. It is painless. Gel is put on your chest, and a metal ball is rolled over it. The machine makes pictures that measure how thick your heart wall is and how much blood your heart is pumping with each heartbeat. If you have a heart murmur, it can tell if the murmur is "innocent" or requires treatment by checking the function of the valves in your heart. It will also detect enlargement of your heart from uncontrolled high blood pressure; that is called *left ventricular hypertrophy* or *LVH*. (See the High Blood Pressure section in this Appendix for more on this.)
- **Cardiac catheterization:** This test is called the "gold standard" for finding out the condition of your coronary arteries. It also can stop heart attacks before they damage your heart muscle if it is performed in time. In this test, which is a type of *angiogram*, a wire is inserted into the large artery in your groin (called the *femoral artery*) and threaded all the way through your body and into your coronary arteries. Dye is injected into your coronary arteries, and pictures are taken that show exactly which arteries are blocked and how badly. If you are having a heart attack, this procedure can clear the blockage, restore blood flow, and prevent permanent damage to your heart muscle. A medical specialist called an *interventional cardiologist* performs this test. The test is invasive (meaning things are poked in you), there are risks, and you have to be sedated while it is done. Not

everyone can have this test, but in certain circumstances it is lifesaving. When your coronary arteries are unblocked during the procedure, it is called *angioplasty*. Sometimes tiny tubes shaped like straws called *stents* are placed in your coronary arteries to keep them open after the procedure.

- **Coronary artery ultrasound:** This test can detect soft plaque that is inside the artery walls and would not be detected with cardiac catheterization alone. This test is done like cardiac catheterization, using a wire that is threaded through your groin into your coronary arteries. This test uses sound waves to make images the same way other ultrasound tests do. The difference in this test is that the probe is *inside* the artery, instead of outside your body as for other ultrasounds. The test is sometimes done with, and has all the same risks as, cardiac catheterization. Unlike a regular cardiac catheterization, the ultrasound can make pictures of the inside of the artery walls and tell how much plaque is present and what type it is.
- **Heart scans—computed tomography (CT) scan and electron beam tomography (EBT) scan:** These are special x-ray tests of your heart that combine the technology of the spiral CT scan (a painless test in which a special CT machine rotates rapidly around your body) along with high-speed, 3D resolution that can construct detailed images of your heart. These tests are used to detect calcium blockages in your coronary arteries. They are sometimes done with dye (contrast) that causes your blood vessels to light up on the images produced, so they are easier to see. These tests have been controversial. The American Heart Association, which was skeptical of them at the beginning, is now recommending them for people with intermediate risks to help determine the extent of blockages. They are noninvasive (unless dye is used), but you do get some radiation as with x-rays. The EBT is considered more accurate and uses less radiation than the CT, but there are far fewer EBT machines around. Unlike cardiac catheterization or coronary ultrasound, no wires are introduced into your body. These tests will not eliminate the need for cardiac catheterization, coronary ultrasound, or both in certain

individuals. They can be good, if expensive, motivational tools that encourage people to change their lifestyles. Getting to see a picture of the blockages already present in the coronary arteries can motivate people to start reducing their risk factors. The scans can cost anywhere from $200 to $700, depending on the type of equipment used.

Medications for Cardiovascular Disease

- **Aspirin:** This is the most commonly used and best-known medicine in the world. It is more than 100 years old. It is widely used; it is potent; it is cheap. It has serious risks and excellent benefits. It is underprescribed by healthcare providers. Aspirin prevents or slows the progression of blood clots that try to form in your heart, brain, or legs. You should only begin taking aspirin under the supervision of a healthcare provider. You should *not* take aspirin if you are allergic, have ulcer disease, have had a recent injury, or are about to have or have recently had surgery.
- **Digoxin:** This drug is given to increase the strength and force of your heartbeat. There has to be a certain amount of it in your blood in order for it to work properly, so you are often given a loading dose (a higher dose) when you first start taking the drug. After that, you must take it regularly and with no skipped doses, or the amount of drug in your blood will drop. Blood tests are required from time to time to make sure there is enough of the drug in your bloodstream for it to be effective. Too much of this drug can slow your heart rate and cause other side effects such as nausea and visual changes.
- **Anti-hypertensive drugs:** We discuss various types of these medications in the High Blood Pressure section in this Appendix. Controlling blood pressure is critical to decreasing the workload of your heart and reducing strain on your blood vessels.
- **Cholesterol-lowering drugs:** We discuss these drugs in the High Cholesterol section in this Appendix. More is being learned about the beneficial effects of these drugs all the time. Statin drugs, in particular, lower cholesterol levels (a risk factor for cardiovascular disease), have anti-inflammatory properties, and seem to make plaques in your arteries more stable. All these effects will lower your

risk from cardiovascular disease.

- **Blood thinners:** Plavix (generic name: clopidogrel), Coumadin (warfarin), and Ticlid (ticlopidine) are examples of blood thinners. Like aspirin, they reduce blood clotting. Sometimes they are used in combination with low-dose aspirin, sometimes not. Do not take aspirin if you are taking one of these drugs without talking to your healthcare provider first.
- **Anti-arrhythmic drugs:** These drugs control irregular heart rhythms. Some are anti-hypertensive drugs, like calcium channel blockers. Others are used to treat cardiovascular emergencies in the hospital, and still others are used under the supervision of a cardiologist.

Resources

American Heart Association
National Center
7272 Greenville Avenue
Dallas, TX 75231
1-800-242-8721
http://www.americanheart.org/

U.S. National Library of Medicine
8600 Rockville Pike
Bethesda, MD 20894
1-888-346-3656
http://www.nlm.nih.gov/

National Stroke Association
9707 East Easter Lane
Centennial, CO 80112
1-800-STROKES
http://www.stroke.org/

Diabetes

Targets

Tests / Measurements	Target Number
Normal fasting blood sugar	< 100 mg / dl
2-hour glucose tolerance test (if non-diabetic)	< 130 mg / dl
Blood sugar before meals (if diabetic)	90 to 130 mg / dl
Blood sugar 2 hours after meals (if diabetic)	< 160 mg / dl
Hemoglobin A1c (HbA1c)	< or = 6.0% - 6.5%
Blood pressure	< or = 120 / 80
Total cholesterol	< 200 mg / dl
LDL cholesterol	< 70 mg / dl
HDL cholesterol	> 50 mg / dl
Triglycerides	< 150 mg / dl
VLDL cholesterol	< 30 mg / dl
Homocysteine	< 10 mmol / L

American Diabetes Association Guidelines http://care.diabetesjournals.org/cgi / content / full / 29 / suppl_1 / s4> and Third Report of the Expert Panel on Detection, Evaluation, and Treatment of High Blood Cholesterol in Adults, Adult Treatment Panel III Guidelines, July 13, 2004. http://www.nhlbi.nih.gov / guidelines / cholesterol / upd-info_prof.htm>

In this table < means less than, and > means greater than.

How to Get to Target

- Lose weight if necessary. Start with a target of losing 10 percent of your current weight. Try to reach BMI of 25 or less.
- Exercise regularly—at least 240 minutes a week at your target heart rate. Start with walking, and ensure that your healthcare provider medically approves your new exercise regimen.
- Eat a low-calorie, low-fat, diabetic diet. Ask your healthcare provider for guidelines.
- Monitor your blood sugar with a home glucose monitor.
- Control your blood pressure.
- Control your cholesterol.
- If you smoke — QUIT!!

Most diabetics will require medication of some sort in conjunction with changes to their lifestyle. If weight loss, diet, and exercise alone, or weight loss, diet, and exercise, plus oral medication, do not control your blood sugar to target, then you will need insulin.

Oral Medications for Diabetes

The following oral medications are routinely prescribed for diabetes. The medications are given with their brand name first (starting with a capital letter) followed by their generic name (all in small letters).

- **Sulfonylureas:** Drugs in this group include *Amaryl/glimepiride, Glucotrol / glipizide, Micronase / glyburide,* and *Diabetal / glyburide.* These drugs work by *stimulating your pancreas to make more insulin.* If you have type 2 diabetes and your body is not sensitive to insulin, you will need more insulin than normal to control your blood sugar. These drugs are usually used in combination with other oral medications. People with sulfa allergies or who are pregnant should not take them. If you are taking this medication, skipping meals or drinking alcohol may cause your blood sugar to become too low (that is, you may get hypoglycemia).
- **Biguanides:** *Glucophage / metformin* is the most common drug in this group. This drug works by *decreasing the amount of glucose made by your liver.* It also *helps your cells become more sensitive to insulin.* It is usually prescribed in combination with other medications. Because much of the glucose in your body comes from food, it is essential that you eat a proper diet in addition to taking this and all diabetes medications.
- **Meglitinides:** Drugs in this group include *Prandin / repaglinide* and *Starlix / nateglinide.* These drugs *increase the amount of insulin made by your pancreas.* They are taken with meals. If taken with sulfonylureas, they can cause your blood sugar to go too low (hypoglycemia).
- **Thiazolidinediones (TZDs):** Drugs in this group include *Avandia / rosiglitazone* and *Actos / pioglitazone.* These drugs are called *insulin sensitizers* because they *both improve insulin insensitivity* and *decrease the amount of glucose made by your liver.* These drugs can *actually stop*

the burnout of beta cells that causes type 2 diabetes *if* they are started early enough. They can *prevent* diabetes if they are started early enough and combined with behavior change (that is, proper diet, weight loss, and exercise). You must have liver function tests when you take these medications because they can cause rare but serious liver problems. In addition to preserving your beta cells, these drugs also help reverse a condition called *fatty liver.* Fatty liver often develops from alcohol abuse and being overweight. It means, literally, fat in your liver. The fat interferes with your liver's ability to function normally, so reversing the condition is a secondary benefit of this group of drugs. These drugs can cause foot or leg swelling, which may be a sign of congestive heart failure (CHF) and so should be reported to your health provider immediately.

- **DPP-4 inhibitors**: *Januvia / sitagliptin phosphate* is the first (but will not be the last) medication in this new type of drug class that was approved by the FDA in October 2006. The drug works by enhancing the body's own ability to lower blood sugar when it is high, particularly after meals. It also decreases the amount of sugar the body makes. Because it only works when blood sugar is high, there is less risk of low blood sugar (hypoglycemia) with this drug than with other types of diabetes medications. It may be used alone or in combination with other diabetes medications.
- **Alpha-glucosidase inhibitors:** Drugs in this group include *Precose / acarbose* and *Glyset / miglitol.* These drugs work *by slowing the breakdown of carbohydr tes in your body and so slowing the rise in blood sugar that occurs after you eat.* They must be taken with the first bite of food. However, they are no substitute for a proper diet. These drugs are less commonly used than the other drugs discussed above.

Just like blood pressure medications, these diabetes medications work in different ways in your body. That means that combinations of these drugs together are usually *more effective than a single drug.*

In addition to medications that lower blood sugars, everyone with diabetes should be on cardio-protective (heart-protecting) medications unless there is some reason you can't take them. Remember, diabetes is a cardiovascular disease risk equivalent (see the Cardiovascular Disease section in this Appendix). That means if you have diabetes, you must pay special attention to protecting your heart and blood vessels by controlling your blood pressure, cholesterol, and other risks for cardiovascular events like heart attacks and stroke. For that reason, everyone with diabetes should also take the following medications.

- **Aspirin:** The recommended dose is 81 mg every day. (See the Cardiovascular Disease section in this Appendix for detailed information on the risks and benefits of aspirin, and who should and shouldn't take it.)
- **ACE inhibitors:** These are blood pressure medications. This particular class of blood pressure medications (along with the **angiotensin II receptor blockers or ARBs**) protect your kidneys from the damage caused by diabetes. Even if your blood pressure is not that high, these medications still protect your kidneys, which are vital target organs. (See the High Blood Pressure section in this Appendix for more on blood pressure medications.)
- **Statins:** These are a type of cholesterol-lowering medication. If you have diabetes, it is important that you keep your cholesterol values to target with aggressive medication treatment, if necessary. (See the High Cholesterol section for detailed information on statins.)
- **Folic acid:** This is a vitamin found in leafy green vegetables, nuts, beans, citrus fruits, fortified breakfast cereals, and some vitamin supplements. Experts believe that if you have diabetes, taking folic acid supplements will reduce your risk of a cardiovascular event (heart attack and stroke). As a supplement at doses of 5 mg per day, it can help treat high homocysteine levels (greater than 10 mmol/L). If your homocysteine level is normal, a dose of 1 mg per day is protective.

Insulin for Diabetes

There are different types of insulin, and they vary by how quickly they start working, how long it takes for them to reach peak effects, and how many hours they keep lowering your blood sugar.

- Rapid and short-acting insulins start lowering blood sugar within 15 to 30 minutes. They are often used in insulin "sliding scales" to control blood sugar that is higher than it should be.

- Medium-acting insulins are usually taken twice a day and last about 12 hours.
- Long-acting insulins last 18 to 24 hours. As of this writing, the newest form of long-acting insulin is called *Lantus* (generic name: *insulin glargine*). It mimics natural insulin and so has no "peak." It is used alone or along with short-acting insulin taken at meals to control your blood sugar evenly and avoid wide swings from high to low.

The preferred approach for insulin administration currently being used is either Lantus alone or a combination of Lantus once a day (usually at night) with *Humalog* (*insulin lispro*), a rapid-acting insulin, which is given 15 minutes before meals and at bedtime as needed. It is administered on sliding-scale doses based on the results of finger-stick blood sugar testing that you do four times a day. *Humalog* not only helps keep your blood sugar to target, but also regulates your glucose metabolism.

The pre-mixed insulins that combine fast-acting and medium-acting insulins together (like 70/30 and 75/25) are falling out of favor because of a gap in the middle of the doses when your blood sugar can rise. There are also insulin pumps available that try to mimic the insulin release that would occur in a non-diabetic. Many diabetics who have their diets well controlled prefer these. New inhaled forms of insulin are just coming on the market at the time of this writing.

The risk with insulin is that your blood sugar can go too low (a condition called *hypoglycemia*). If you take too much insulin, don't eat enough food, or both, your blood sugar may drop so low that you become confused or even unconscious. This is very dangerous. If you are driving or alone, and there is no one there to get sugar into you, you can die.

Your Diet

Whether you take oral medication, insulin, or both, you will discover that successful control of your diabetes depends on what you eat. The proper foods, in the proper amounts, at the proper times will do more to control your blood sugars than anything else you do.

Many new diabetics hope that their medications will control their blood sugar so they won't have to pay attention to their diet. Unfortunately, it doesn't work this way. As long as your diet is out of control, your blood sugar will be, too. Combining diet and medications to control your blood sugar requires knowledge and desire, but it can be done. Once your blood sugar is under control, you will feel better and find that the lifestyle required isn't as hard as you first thought.

Diabetic Risks

Diabetes is a complicated disease that you can't just forget about. If you do, you will certainly face some of the risks outlined below.

- Birth defects in newborns or overly large infants
- Blindness
- Cardiovascular disease
- Carpal tunnel syndrome
- Erectile dysfunction
- Fungal and bacterial infections
- Heart attack
- High blood pressure
- Impaired digestion
- Kidney disease
- Loss of toes, feet, or legs
- Neuropathy (nerve damage)
- Peripheral vascular disease
- Poor wound healing
- Stroke (brain attack)
- Tooth and gum disease

Checklist for Diabetics — Getting the Care You Need

☐ I understand my treatment plan. I understand what I have been instructed to do and why.

☐ I know the goal of treatment. (**It's tight blood sugar control!**)

☐ I know that tight blood sugar control will help prevent damage to my heart, brain, kidneys, and nerves.

☐ I know that tight blood sugar control will prolong the length and quality of my life.

- ☐ My healthcare provider started me on medication, a diabetic diet, and a weight loss program early in the course of my disease.
- ☐ I completely understand the ADA (American Diabetes Association) diet. I know how to design a meal plan of foods I enjoy, and I am following it strictly.
- ☐ I exercise at least 240 minutes per week at my target heart rate.
- ☐ If my BMI is over 25, I am working on or have reduced my weight by 10 percent of my total weight.
- ☐ I know when and how to take my medications, and I take them exactly as ordered. I know what side effects to be alert for, and I know when I should contact my provider for follow-up tests and checkups.
- ☐ I am taking a daily aspirin (if I am not allergic or have stomach problems that prevent me from taking aspirin).
- ☐ I am taking a medication called an ACE inhibitor or ARB that is protecting my heart and kidneys and controlling my blood pressure.
- ☐ My provider examines my feet for problems each visit.
- ☐ I inspect my feet daily and call my provider as soon as I find any blisters, cuts, or ulcers.
- ☐ I have reached my target hemoglobin A1c (6.0 to 6.5 percent), and I get it measured every three months.
- ☐ I have reached my target blood pressure of less than 120 / 80 mm Hg.
- ☐ I have reached my target LDL cholesterol of less than 70 mg / dl.
- ☐ I have reached my target HDL cholesterol of greater than 50 mg / dl if I am male; greater than 55 mg / dl if I am female.
- ☐ I self-monitor my blood sugar as often as my provider recommends; I keep a record of the dates and times of all my blood sugar readings; and I take my records with me to each appointment with my provider.

When I self-monitor my blood sugars:

- ☐ My fasting blood sugars are less than 100 mg / dl.
- ☐ My blood sugars that I check two hours after meals are less than 160 mg / dl.
- ☐ My bedtime blood sugar is between 100 and 160 mg / dl.

- ☐ I know how to handle diabetic complications or special situations like illness and low blood sugar (hypoglycemia).
- ☐ I know when and how often to see my healthcare provider for checkups.
- ☐ I know I am responsible for managing my diabetes.
- ☐ I have received referrals to and have followed up as needed with specialists such as diabetes educators, licensed dieticians, podiatrists (foot doctors), ophthalmologists (eye doctors), dentists, exercise physiologists, and, as needed, mental health professionals to help me educate and care for myself and my diabetes.

I keep written records with dates and times of the following:

- ☐ The medications I take (including the doses).
- ☐ My diet (counting carbohydrate grams and calories).
- ☐ My body weight.
- ☐ My physical activities (number of minutes of exercise and heart rate during exercise).
- ☐ Any signs and symptoms of high or low blood sugar I have.
- ☐ I review my written records with my provider at regular intervals.
- ☐ I am satisfied that I am knowledgeable and can handle my diabetes in partnership with my provider.

Resources

American Diabetes Association
ATTN: National Call Center
1701 North Beauregard Street
Alexandria, VA 22311
1-800-DIABETES
(1-800-342-2383)
http://www.diabetes.org/

Diabetic Diet Information
Nutrition & Recipes
American Diabetes Association
http://www.diabetes.org/nutrition-and-recipes/nutrition/overview.jsp

Blood Sugar Record

Date	Time	Blood Sugar	Medication or Insulin Taken

Metabolic Syndrome

If you have any three of the following five factors, you have the condition called metabolic syndrome.

- **Central obesity.** That means being overweight, with a BMI greater than 25, and carrying your fat in your abdomen. A waist girth greater than 35 inches in women and greater than 40 inches in men is considered central obesity.
- **High fasting triglycerides** (greater than 150 mg / dl).
- **Low HDL cholesterol** (less than 50 mg / dl in women and less than 40 mg / dl in men).
- **High blood pressure** (measurements greater than 130 / 85 mm Hg) or taking medication for high blood pressure even if your pressure is under control.
- **Fasting blood glucose** (sugar) greater than 110 mg / dl.

Targets

Tests / Measurements	Target Number
BMI	< or = 25
Waist circumference	< 35 inches in women and < 40 inches in men
Triglycerides	< 150 mg / dl
HDL cholesterol	> 50 mg / dl in women and > 40 mg / dl in men
Blood pressure	< 130 / 80 mm Hg
Fasting blood sugar	< 100 mg / dl

Third Report of the Expert Panel on Detection, Evaluation, and Treatment of High Blood Cholesterol in Adults, Adult Treatment Panel III Guidelines, July 13, 2004. (http://www.nhlbi.nih.gov/guidelines/cholesterol/upd-info_prof.htm)

In this table < means less than and > means greater than.

Medications for Metabolic Syndrome

Your healthcare provider can determine if you have metabolic syndrome from routine blood tests. The best treatment is *changing your lifestyle*. However, the following medications should be taken to reach targets.

- **Aspirin:** If you are not allergic to aspirin and do not have ulcers, taking 81 mg of aspirin each day helps prevent blood clots that can lead to heart attack and stroke. Check with your healthcare provider before starting this or any other new medications. Also, because aspirin is a blood thinner, you should stop taking it a day or two before you have any kind of surgery. Always include aspirin in your list of medications that you show to your providers.
- **Folic acid:** If your homocysteine level is greater than 10 mmol / L , you should be taking folic acid supplements at a dose of 5 mg per day. This is a prescription-strength dose that you can get from your healthcare provider. You should also try to get more folic acid in the foods you eat. Foods rich in folic acid include enriched, fortified cereals, enriched whole-grain breads, and leafy, dark green vegetables.
- **Blood pressure medications:** See the High Blood Pressure section in this Appendix.
- **Cholesterol-lowering medications:** See the High Cholesterol section in this Appendix.
- **Diabetes medications:** See the Diabetes section in this Appendix.

Resources

Third Report of the Expert Panel on Detection, Evaluation, and Treatment of High Blood Cholesterol in Adults
http://www.nhlbi.nih.gov/guidelines/cholesterol/

American Heart Association
National Center
7272 Greenville Avenue
Dallas, TX 75231
1-800-242-8721
http://www.americanheart.org/presenter.jhtml?identifier=4756

U.S. National Library of Medicine
8600 Rockville Pike
Bethesda, MD 20894
1-888-346-3656
http://www.nlm.nih.gov/medlineplus/metabolicsyndrome.html

High Blood Pressure

Target

Your optimal target blood pressure is a systolic blood pressure (top number) of 120 mm Hg or lower and a diastolic blood pressure (bottom number) of 80 mm Hg or lower.

Measurements	**Systolic Blood Pressure**	**Diastolic Blood Pressure**
Normal blood pressure target	< 120	< 80
Abnormal blood pressure		
Prehypertension	120 to 139	80 to 89
Stage 1 high blood pressure	140 to 159	90 to 99
Stage 2 high blood pressure	> 160	> 100

Seventh Report of the Joint National Committee on Prevention, Detection, Evaluation and Treatment of High Blood Pressure (http://www.nhlbi.nih.gov/guidelines/hypertension/index.htm)

Values are in mm Hg.

In this table, < means less than and > means greater than.

Tests

The danger of uncontrolled blood pressure is from the damage it does to your vital organs like your heart, kidneys, and blood vessels in your eyes. Your healthcare provider may order the following tests to check for damage.

- **Echocardiography:** This test checks the pumping ability, shape, and size of your heart. It uses sound waves to produce images of your heart muscles and valves. It is painless. A metal ball is used as a sensor and rolled over a gel that has been put on your chest. The machine uses the sound waves to create images that measure how thick your heart wall is, how much blood your heart is pumping with each heartbeat, and because it checks the valves of the heart, it can determine whether a heart murmur (if you have one) is innocent or requires treatment. When you have high blood pressure, your heart muscle must pump against high pressure all the time, so your heart (just like any other muscle) becomes enlarged. This is called *left ventricular hypertrophy*, or *LVH*. It is a sign of target organ damage from your high blood pressure. LVH can be a precursor to congestive heart failure (CHF), which occurs when your heart tires out and gradually loses its ability to pump enough blood to your body. LVH is treated with medications and can sometimes even be reversed (this is called *remodeling*).

- **A urine test for microalbuminuria:** This test checks to see if you have a microscopic amount of protein in your urine. This is an early sign of kidney damage from high blood pressure. The presence of any protein in your urine is an abnormal finding. People with high blood pressure can have protein in their urine because of the high pressure under which the blood is pushed through their kidneys. Your kidneys are complicated organs, and one way they work is to filter the blood that is pumped through them. You can think of the filtering process in your kidneys like the actions of a fishing net. If there are holes in the net, the fish can swim through. High blood pressure pushes your blood so forcefully through your kidneys that it tears holes in the net, so the protein (fish) gets through and spills into your urine. By the time protein shows up in a regular urine test, it is way too high. The test for microalbuminuria detects the problem much, much earlier. The treatment is control of your blood pressure to target.
- **A dilated eye exam by an eye doctor:** This exam will detect damage to the blood vessels of your retina that can be caused by high blood pressure. Seeing an eye doctor every year isn't just about telling if you need glasses or having your glasses changed. It is an important medical examination that can detect and treat damage to your eyes from a number of health risks before they cause permanent loss of your vision.

Medications for High Blood Pressure

If you are unable to control your blood pressure to target with lifestyle changes alone, you need medication. Most people require combinations of *more than one medication* to control their blood pressure adequately, and many need *as many as four medications*. Current guidelines recommend that your healthcare provider should treat your high blood pressure aggressively to get you to target. You will benefit from taking as many medications as necessary to reach blood pressure goals. Remember, the evil is the high blood pressure—*not* the medications that treat it.

- Blood pressure medications work in different ways, and the reason more than one is required is that a combination is often more effective than a single drug. Medications below are listed by both their brand names (starting in capital letters) and their generic names (in all small letters). These are the eight main types of blood pressure medications, with examples of some of the commonly prescribed drugs.
- **Diuretics:** Drugs in this group include *Lasix / furosemide, Maxzide / hydrochlorothiazide , HCTZ or HCT, Bumex / bumetanide, Demadex / torsemide, Aldactone / spironolactone,* and *Zaroxolyn / metolazone.* These are "water pills." They increase urination and should be taken in the morning so as not to disturb your sleep. They get rid of excess fluid and decrease your circulating blood volume, thereby lowering blood pressure. Sodium (salt) draws water into your blood vessels, increasing circulating blood volume and so increasing blood pressure. That is why a low-sodium diet helps lower blood pressure. A low-sodium diet, in combination with a diuretic, can be very effective in lowering blood pressure in some individuals. Some diuretics cause loss of potassium, while others do not. Discuss with your healthcare provider whether you need to take potassium supplements along with your diuretic. Do **not** take potassium supplements unless instructed to do so. Too much potassium can be dangerous and cause heart problems. So can too little potassium.
- **ACE inhibitors:** Drugs in this group include *Accupril / quinapril, Monopril / fosinopril, Prinivil and Zestril / lisinopril, Vasotec / enalapril, Altace / ramipril, Capoten / captopril, Lotensin / benazepril, Mavik / trandolapril,* and *Univasc / moexipril.* These drugs block a naturally occurring chemical in your body called *angiotensin-converting enzyme* (ACE). This chemical causes blood vessels to constrict (get narrower) and so it increases blood pressure. By blocking (inhibiting) this chemical, blood vessel constriction doesn't occur, vessels stay relaxed, and blood pressure is lower as a result. These drugs also

protect your kidneys and are useful for people who have both diabetes and high blood pressure.

- **Angiotensin II receptor blockers (ARBs):** Drugs in this group include *Cozaar / losartan, Diovan / valsartan, Avapro / irbesartan, Atacand / candesartan, Benicar / olmesartan, Micardis / telmisartan,* and *Teveten / eprosartan.* These drugs work in a similar way to ACE inhibitors, but they have a slightly different biochemistry. People who have the side effect of a cough with ACE inhibitors can often take these drugs without getting that unpleasant effect. Like ACE inhibitors, these drugs protect your kidneys. They also are good for people with diabetes.
- **Direct renin inhibitor:** This is a new class of blood pressure medication that came on the market in 2007. The only drug currently available in this class is *Tekturna / aliskiren*. It inhibits a kidney enzyme called renin that is involved with the regulation of blood pressure. It works earlier in the same chemical pathway as the ACE inhibitors and ARBs listed above and is sometimes combined with diuretics.
- **Beta-blockers:** Drugs in this group include *Inderal / propranolol, Lopressor and Toprol / metoprolol, Tenormin / atenolol,* and *Betapace / sotalol.* These drugs decrease the rate and force of your heartbeat and dilate (relax) the vessels around your heart. Some constrict your peripheral blood vessels. Decreasing the output from your heart lowers your blood pressure, and relaxing the vessels around your heart improves blood flow and thereby the flow of oxygen to your heart. Because these drugs decrease the heart's workload, they are often prescribed after a person has a heart attack.
- **Calcium channel blockers:** Drugs in this group include *Calan, Covera, Isoptin,* and *Verelan / verapamil; Norvasc / amlodipine; Cardizem, Diltia XT, Cartia XT, Dilacor XR, Tiazac / diltiazem; Adalat* and *Procardia / nifedipine;* and *Dynacirc CR / isradipine.* These drugs block the exchange of calcium between your cells and your blood, both in your heart and in your peripheral circulation. This stops the constriction of your blood vessels that would normally occur, thereby lowering your blood pressure. These drugs are particularly good for people who get angina or coronary artery spasm because they control both blood

pressure and chest pain.

- **Alpha-adrenergic blockers:** Drugs in this group include *Catapress / clonidine, Cardura / doxazosin, Hytrin / terazosin, Minipress / prazosin,* and *Wytensin / guanabenz.* Alpha adrenergic receptors are part of your nervous system and are located all over your body, including in your blood vessels. When they are stimulated, they cause constriction of your blood vessels; as a result, your blood pressure rises. These drugs block the receptors so that they don't constrict; as a result, your blood pressure stays lower. Side effects include dizziness and low blood pressure that can occur with sudden changes in position, such as standing up quickly. These drugs are helpful in men with enlarged prostates because they make it easier to urinate. If you have prostate enlargement and high blood pressure, these blockers might be a good medication for you.
- **Combination alpha- and beta-blockers:** Drugs in this group include *Coreg / carvedilol* and *Normodyne / labetalol.* These drugs act on *both* the beta receptors (to decrease your heart's workload and increase the circulation to your heart) *and* the alpha receptors (to prevent vasoconstriction in the peripheral bloods vessels located in places like your hands and feet). They often are used for people who have congestive heart failure. They also are used in people who have an enlarged heart from high blood pressure (*left ventricular hypertrophy* or *LVH*) and can actually remodel or reverse some of the heart damage caused by uncontrolled blood pressure.

If you have high blood pressure, you must be careful of the over-the-counter medications. Many increase your blood pressure—some to possibly dangerous levels. Pharmacies are filled with remedies you can buy without a prescription, and many are not safe if you have high blood pressure. Check with your healthcare provider or pharmacist about any over-the-counter medication you are considering taking.

Resources

The Seventh Report of the Joint National Committee on Prevention, Detection, Evaluation, and Treatment of High Blood Pressure
http://www.nhlbi.nih.gov/guidelines/hypertension/

National Heart, Lung, and Blood Institute (NHLBI)
NHLBI Health Information Center
Attention: Web Site
P.O. Box 30105
Bethesda, MD 20824
1-301-592-8573
http://www.nhlbi.nih.gov/

National Heart, Lung, and Blood Institute (NHLBI)
DASH Eating Plan
http://www.nhlbi.nih.gov/health/public/heart/hbp/dash/introduction.html

Blood Pressure Record

Date	Time	Blood Pressure

Check your blood pressure morning and evening if your blood pressure is uncontrolled or you are taking new medication.

High Cholesterol

Targets

The goals and targets for cholesterol treatment keep evolving. The best target numbers to reach for are under ongoing study by medical experts. In addition, the lipoprotein tests described below that measure cholesterol particle sizes are also under discussion as screening tools.

The targets given below are from guidelines endorsed by the National Heart, Lung, and Blood Institute; the American College of Cardiology Foundation; and the American Heart Association, and are current at the time of this writing. These targets are revised periodically based on ongoing research in preventing disease caused by high cholesterol. The targets keep getting lowered. Experts aren't sure how low cholesterol should be, but at present they believe the lower, the better for everyone—regardless of other risks. Stay tuned for further information and research. (You can check for updates on the Internet or from your healthcare provider.) In the meantime —how low can you go?

There are four numbers in a standard cholesterol profile:

- **Total cholesterol** is a combination of all the types of cholesterol in your body.
- **LDL (low-density lipoprotein) cholesterol** is the "bad" cholesterol.
- **HDL (high-density lipoprotein) cholesterol** is the "good" cholesterol.
- **Triglycerides** are fats that circulate around in your blood; they also increase your heart attack and stroke risk.

Your healthcare provider may also measure your level of **VLDL (very low density lipoprotein) cholesterol.** That is the "very bad" cholesterol because it works its way easily inside the walls of your blood vessels to cause plaque.

Targets

Tests / Measurements	Target Number
Total cholesterol	< 200 mg / dl
LDL cholesterol*	< 70 mg / dl
HDL cholesterol	> 50 mg / dl
Triglycerides	< 150 mg / dl
VLDL cholesterol	< 30 mg / dl

Third Report of the Expert Panel on Detection, Evaluation, and Treatment of High Blood Cholesterol in Adults, Adult Treatment Panel III Guidelines, July 13, 2004. (http://www.nhlbi.nih.gov / guidelines / cholesterol / upd-info_prof.htm)

**Determining your target LDL depends on your other risk factors (discussed below).*

In this table < means less than and > means greater than.

How to Determine Your Target LDL

Your target LDL cholesterol depends on whether or not you have coronary heart disease (CHD), which means a prior heart attack or known coronary artery disease or any CHD risk equivalents. CHD equivalents are diabetes, peripheral vascular disease, abdominal aortic aneurysm, carotid artery disease, and metabolic syndrome.

- If you have CHD or a CHD risk equivalent, your LDL target is **less than 70 mg / dl**. You should take medication if your LDL is not to target.
- If you have two or more of the following risk factors—high blood pressure, smoking, HDL less than 40 mg / dl, a family history of heart disease, or if you are a man over 45 or a woman over 55—your LDL target is **less than 100 mg / dl.** (Note: If your HDL is greater than 60 mg / dl, you may subtract one other risk factor.) Your healthcare provider *may* advise that you take medication if your LDL is between 100 and 130 mg / dl to further lower your risk.
- If you have no CHD, no CHD risk equivalents, and fewer than two of the risks factors listed in the second category (above), your LDL target is less than 160 mg / dl (but less than 130 to 100 mg / dl is better).

Lipoprotein Test

The standard cholesterol test is still a simple blood test that gives the above information. However, there are new tests for cholesterol called *lipoprotein tests* that measure not only the *amount* of the different types of cholesterol, but also their *size*. As of this writing, neither the American Heart

Association nor the National Institutes of Health have recommended them as screening tests. They are expensive and cost about $100. Healthcare providers are still divided about the necessity of adding more expensive tests to the medical evaluation of high cholesterol. But these tests have proven popular with the public. Some people find that seeing their results helps motivate them to get healthier. Lipoprotein tests will certainly be more widely used in the future. So what's so different about lipoprotein testing compared with standard cholesterol testing?

Lipoproteins are the protein particles that carry cholesterol and triglycerides. *The number, size, and type of lipoproteins a person has are a better predictor of cardiovascular disease risk than cholesterol levels alone.*

For example, even people with normal cholesterol levels can be at increased risk for heart attack and stroke if they have high levels of the LDL and VLDL lipoproteins. Conversely, if they have very high levels of HDL lipoprotein, they may have less risk even if their total cholesterol is high.

Size matters where lipoproteins are concerned, and lipoprotein testing measures the size of the particles.

- Large HDL particles remove cholesterol from your arteries; small HDL particles do not.
- LDL particles comes in three sizes—all bad. The smallest LDL is thought to be the most dangerous. Small LDLs penetrate your artery walls more easily than large LDLs and become trapped there, where their cholesterol can be released, causing plaque to build up.
- Large VLDL particles are the most dangerous and are most affected by how much fat you eat.

Based on this information, a combination of increased numbers of both *large* VLDL and *small* HDL may place you at much greater risk for heart disease.

The following people might benefit from lipoprotein testing:

- Those trying to prevent heart disease.
- Those who have a high-risk family history of heart disease.
- Those who have metabolic syndrome.
- Those who have heart disease but have few risk factors they can change.

- Those who wish to monitor the effectiveness of risk reduction efforts like weight loss or exercise.
- Those who want to monitor the effectiveness of their medications.

If you think you would like lipoprotein testing, check with your insurance company to see if the testing is covered and discuss your interest with your healthcare provider.

Getting to Target

Many people are unable to reach target cholesterol levels with lifestyle changes alone. If it is your genes rather than your lifestyle that is causing your high cholesterol, you will need medication *plus* lifestyle changes to reach your goal. If you have fewer than two risk factors and have just discovered that your cholesterol is elevated, a 12-week trial of lifestyle changes is a reasonable approach to see if you can reach target numbers without medication.

If you have known CHD or a CHD risk equivalent (described previously) *and* you have high cholesterol, you should take medication. And, if you do need cholesterol medication, you will probably need to keep taking it for life. If you reach target numbers with medication and then stop taking it, your cholesterol numbers will likely rise again. Never forget that the evil is the high cholesterol numbers—not the medications that lower them.

Medications for High Cholesterol

The following medications are used to lower cholesterol levels. They are given with their brand name (starting with a capital letter) followed by their generic name (in all small letters).

Statins

Drugs in this group include *Lipitor / atorvastatin, Zocor / simvastatin, Pravachol / pravastatin, Mevacor / lovastatin, Lescol / fluvastatin,* and *Crestor / rosuvastatin.*

Statins are the most commonly prescribed drugs and the first-line treatments for high cholesterol. They lower total cholesterol and LDL, and they raise HDL—all the desired effects. Statins may have other beneficial effects, too; possible effects still under study are improved bone density in women, reduced irregular heart rhythms, reduced incidence of stroke, reduced development of diabetes, and reduced dementia in older adults.

These medicines should be taken on a full stomach, preferably after your evening meal, as this is when your body produces the most cholesterol. Try to take this medication separately from other medications so that it can be absorbed more fully.

All people who take statins should have a cholesterol profile and liver function tests *before starting the medication*. The liver function tests are also done regularly *while you are taking the medication*. Your healthcare provider checks your liver function because statins are metabolized by your liver. (Liver function tests are the ALT and AST blood tests. For more on these tests, see Routine Laboratory Tests in this Appendix.)

Statins are safe for most people, and side effects are rare. Occasionally, there is some mild stomach upset that usually goes away after a couple of days. Sometimes people experience mild muscle aches (called *myalgia*) that can often be managed by taking CoQ10 supplements, 150 mg twice a day. *Very rarely,* taking statins can cause a serious side effect of severe muscle pain and dark-colored urine that, if left untreated and the drug is not stopped, can lead to a life-threatening condition called *rhabdomyolysis.*

To put things in perspective, according to a joint report by the American College of Cardiology; American Heart Association; and National Heart, Lung, and Blood Institute, fatal rhabdomyolysis occurs in only about one in one million prescriptions. That means it is *very rare* and it is *not* a reason to be afraid of the drug. The report further states, *"There is a well-documented under-use of statins in clinical practice. Statins have proven to be extremely safe in the vast majority of patients receiving them."*

If you are prescribed a statin, report any muscle pain or dark-colored urine to your healthcare provider immediately so that he or she can advise you.

The following people are at higher risk for getting side effects from statins:

- Older adults, particularly those over 80.
- Women more than men.
- People who are frail and have a small body frame.
- People with kidney disease, diabetes, or alcoholism.

- People who drink large quantities of grapefruit juice (a quart or more per day).

The following drugs increase the risk of side effects if you take them with statins:

- *Lopid / gemfibrozil* taken with statins is potentially dangerous (caution should be taken with other fibrates, too, but *Tricor / fenofibrate* and *Antara / miconrized senofibrate* are the safest if carefully monitored by your healthcare provider).
- Generic *cyclosporine* (brand names: *Sandimmune* and *Neoral).*
- Generic *itraconazole (Sporanox)* and *ketoconazole (Nizoral).*
- Generic *erythromycin* and *clarithromycin (Biaxin).*
- HIV protease inhibitors.
- Generic *nefazodone* (an anti-depressant).
- Generic *verapamil* (brand names: *Calan, Covera, Isoptin, Verelan*).
- Generic *diltiazem* (brand names: *Cardizem, Dilacor XR, Tiazac*).
- Generic *amiodarone* (brand names: *Cordarone, Pacerone*).

Cholesterol absorption inhibitor

The only drug in this group as of this writing is *Zetia / ezetimibe.* This medication has been on the market since October of 2002. It is the first drug of its class. It can be used alone but is most effective in combination with other cholesterol-lowering drugs, particularly statins. Zetia works by stopping the absorption of cholesterol in your small intestine. It blocks the cholesterol from food as well as your body's own cholesterol that has been made by your liver and secreted in your bile. Zetia can be taken at any time of the day and does not need to be taken with food or meals. The drug is activated by your liver, so just as with statin therapy, you must have regular blood tests to check your liver function. Report any muscle aches immediately to your healthcare provider. Zetia is combined with the statin *Zocor / simvastatin* in the combination drug *Vytorin.*

Fibrates

Drugs in this group include *Lopid / gemfibrozil, Tricor / fenofibrate,* and *Antara / micronized sansfibrate.* These medications are used in people with high triglyceride levels. Generally, statins and fibrates are not used together. If they are, it is with caution and close monitoring with liver function tests.

Lopid should not be taken with statins, while Tricor and Antara are used together with statins for people with both high cholesterol and high triglycerides.

Omega-3 fish oils

The only pharmaceutical fish oil on the market was called Omacor but its name was changed to Lovaza. Omega-3 supplements can also be purchased in the health food stores. Omega-3 fish oils are known to lower cholesterol, particularly triglycerides. Omega-3s are found in fatty fish such as salmon, mackerel, lake trout, sardines, and herring. They can also be obtained in dietary supplements. The American Heart Association recommends consuming fatty fish twice a week, taking 1 gram of fish oils per day if you have cardiovascular disease, and taking 2 to 4 grams per day if you have high triglycerides.

Resins

Drugs in this group include *Welchol / colesevelam* and *Questran / cholestyramine*. These medications are used to lower total cholesterol and high LDL cholesterol. They have little effect on triglycerides and may even raise them. Resins act by binding bile acids, resulting in a decreased cholesterol production and thereby lowering your cholesterol levels. These medications should be taken 1 to 2 hours before or 4 to 6 hours after other medications because they will bind the other medications and prevent them from being absorbed. Also, they should be taken just before or with meals. The main side effects of these medications are constipation and bloating. These side effects usually subside once your body has time to get used to the medication. Drink more fluids and eat more fiber to prevent constipation.

Niacin

An example of a brand name for niacin is *Niaspan*. Niacin is a vitamin and is used in addition to other cholesterol medications. It is helpful in lowering high triglycerides and raising HDL (the "good" cholesterol). People taking niacin must have regular blood tests to check their liver function. In rare cases, you may have to stop taking it if your liver function becomes abnormal. Niacin should be taken whole—do not crush or chew it. Take it at bedtime with a low-fat snack. Do not drink alcohol or hot beverages at the time you take niacin, because they increase the chances that you will get side effects. Be careful of vitamin supplements with large doses of niacin in them as this may also increase your chance of side effects. The common side effects include flushing, itching, and headache. These can be controlled by taking 325 mg of aspirin or a non-steroidal anti-inflammatory (like Advil or Aleve) 30 minutes before you take the niacin. If the itching is persistent, take an antihistamine (like Benadryl).

Resources

Third Report of the Expert Panel on Detection, Evaluation, and Treatment of High Blood Cholesterol in Adults
http://www.nhlbi.nih.gov/guidelines/cholesterol/

The National Heart, Lung, and Blood Institute (NHLBI)
NHLBI Health Information Center
Attention: Web Site
P.O. Box 30105
Bethesda, MD 20824
1-301-592-8573
http://www.nhlbi.nih.gov/

Weight

Targets

Body Mass Index (BMI) measures your body fat based on both your weight and your height. Research has shown that your health risks increase when your BMI is greater than 25. For that reason, a BMI of less than 25 is our target for reducing health risks from excess weight. However, if a BMI that low is not reasonable for you, don't stop trying to lose weight. Losing 10 percent to 15 percent of your total body weight will pay huge health benefits and will dramatically improve your life and reduce your health risks.

Measurements	**BMI**
Underweight	< 18.5
Normal weight target	18.5 to 24.9
Overweight	25.0 to 29.9
Obesity	30.0 to 39.9
Morbid obesity	> 40.0

In this table < means less than and > means greater than.

Waist measurement determines central obesity, a known risk factor for cardiovascular disease. (See the Metabolic Syndrome section in this Appendix for more.)

	Waist Measurement in Inches
Women's target	< 35
Men's target	< 40

Waist / hip ratio is another risk factor for cardiovascular disease. To find yours, take your waist measurement in inches and divide it by your hip measurement in inches.

	Waist / Hip Ratio
Women's target	< 0.8
Men's target	< 0.9

BMI (Body Mass Index) Table

Body Mass Index Table

	Normal						Overweight					Obese										Extreme Obesity														
BMI	19	20	21	22	23	24	25	26	27	28	29	30	31	32	33	34	35	36	37	38	39	40	41	42	43	44	45	46	47	48	49	50	51	52	53	54
Height (inches)	Body Weight (pounds)																																			
58	91	96	100	105	110	115	119	124	129	134	138	143	148	153	158	162	167	172	177	181	186	191	196	201	205	210	215	220	224	229	234	239	244	248	253	258
59	94	99	104	109	114	119	124	128	133	138	143	148	153	158	163	168	173	178	183	188	193	198	203	208	212	217	222	227	232	237	242	247	252	257	262	267
60	97	102	107	112	118	123	128	133	138	143	148	153	158	163	168	174	179	184	189	194	199	204	209	215	220	225	230	235	240	245	250	255	261	266	271	276
61	100	106	111	116	122	127	132	137	143	148	153	158	164	169	174	180	185	190	195	201	206	211	217	222	227	232	238	243	248	254	259	264	269	275	280	285
62	104	109	115	120	126	131	136	142	147	153	158	164	169	175	180	186	191	196	202	207	213	218	224	229	235	240	246	251	256	262	267	273	278	284	289	295
63	107	113	118	124	130	135	141	146	152	158	163	169	175	180	186	191	197	203	208	214	220	225	231	237	242	248	254	259	265	270	278	282	287	293	299	304
64	110	116	122	128	134	140	145	151	157	163	169	174	180	186	192	197	204	209	215	221	227	232	238	244	250	256	262	267	273	279	285	291	296	302	308	314
65	114	120	126	132	138	144	150	156	162	168	174	180	186	192	198	204	210	216	222	228	234	240	246	252	258	264	270	276	282	288	294	300	306	312	318	324
66	118	124	130	136	142	148	155	161	167	173	179	186	192	198	204	210	216	223	229	235	241	247	253	260	266	272	278	284	291	297	303	309	315	322	328	334
67	121	127	134	140	146	153	159	166	172	178	185	191	198	204	211	217	223	230	236	242	249	255	261	268	274	280	287	293	299	306	312	319	325	331	338	344
68	125	131	138	144	151	158	164	171	177	184	190	197	203	210	216	223	230	236	243	249	256	262	269	276	282	289	295	302	308	315	322	328	335	341	348	354
69	128	135	142	149	155	162	169	176	182	189	196	203	209	216	223	230	236	243	250	257	263	270	277	284	291	297	304	311	318	324	331	338	345	351	358	365
70	132	139	146	153	160	167	174	181	188	195	202	209	216	222	229	236	243	250	257	264	271	278	285	292	299	306	313	320	327	334	341	348	355	362	369	376
71	136	143	150	157	165	172	179	186	193	200	208	215	222	229	236	243	250	257	265	272	279	286	293	301	308	315	322	329	338	343	351	358	365	372	379	386
72	140	147	154	162	169	177	184	191	199	206	213	221	228	235	242	250	258	265	272	279	287	294	302	309	316	324	331	338	346	353	361	368	375	383	390	397
73	144	151	159	166	174	182	189	197	204	212	219	227	235	242	250	257	265	272	280	288	295	302	310	318	325	333	340	348	355	363	371	378	386	393	401	408
74	148	155	163	171	179	186	194	202	210	218	225	233	241	249	256	264	272	280	287	295	303	311	319	326	334	342	350	358	365	373	381	389	396	404	412	420
75	152	160	168	176	184	192	200	208	216	224	232	240	248	256	264	272	279	287	295	303	311	319	327	335	343	351	359	367	375	383	391	399	407	415	423	431
76	156	164	172	180	189	197	205	213	221	230	238	246	254	263	271	279	287	295	304	312	320	328	336	344	353	361	369	377	385	394	402	410	418	426	435	443

Source: Adapted from *Clinical Guidelines on the Identification, Evaluation, and Treatment of Overweight and Obesity in Adults: The Evidence Report.*

Calculating BMI

Formula: (Weight [pounds] / Height^2 [in inches]) x 703

When using a handheld calculator, if your calculator has a square function, divide your weight (in pounds) by your height (in inches) squared, multiply by 703, and round to one decimal place.

*Or **calculate: (Weight [pounds] / Height [inches]) / Height [inches]) x 703***

If your calculator does not have a square function, divide your weight by your height twice, multiply by 703, and round to one decimal place.

Medications for Weight Loss

Medication is rarely appropriate for weight loss. It should only be used under the supervision of a healthcare provider in conjunction with a comprehensive weight loss program that includes a healthy diet and an exercise program. For certain high-risk individuals—those with BMIs greater than 30 and no other weight-related risk factors or diseases, or those with BMIs greater than 27 plus weight-related risk factors or diseases—two drugs are currently approved by the Food and Drug Administration for long-term treatment of obesity. They are given with their brand name (starting with a capital letter) followed by their generic name (in all small letters).

- ***Xenical / orlistat:*** This medication works by reducing fat absorption in your gastrointestinal tract. Because it reduces fat absorption, it interferes with the absorption of fat-soluble vitamins (A, D, E, and beta-carotene) as well. This medication can have unpleasant side effects, particularly if you eat a high-fat diet. These include nausea, vomiting, abdominal pain, oily spotting, and fatty oily stool. However, for obese people with metabolic syndrome, this medication reduces their risk factors for coronary heart disease. In one study of this medication in diabetics, after one year of treatment, the orlistat group lost 6.2 percent of their body weight and the group taking a placebo (a pill that had no drug in it) lost 4.3 percent of their body weight. As you can see, the weight loss when taking this drug is not dramatic, so it is recommended only for people who have severe obesity and who are at high risk for premature cardiac death. *Orlistat* is now available as an over-the-counter medicine named "Alli."

- ***Meridia / sibutramine:*** This medication works in your brain to suppress your appetite. This medication can cause a significant increase in blood pressure, so you may not be able to take it if you have high blood pressure. If you do take it, your blood pressure should be checked regularly. Side effects include dry mouth, headache, constipation, insomnia, and decreased appetite. Because of the appetite-suppressing effects, sibutramine promotes weight loss in conjunction with a healthy diet and exercise. If you are taking an anti-depressant or other medications that also act in the brain, you may not be able to take this medication.

Behavior change that includes proper diet and adequate exercise is the best treatment for reducing your weight and controlling your other risks.

Medications are rarely indicated for weight loss.

Resources

Clinical Guidelines on the Identification, Evaluation, and Treatment of Overweight and Obesity in Adults
National Heart, Lung, and Blood Institute (NHLBI)
http://www.nhlbi.nih.gov/guidelines/obesity/ob_home.htm

Food Diary

Day			Date					
Food	Portion Size	Calories	Fat 30%	Cholesterol < 300 mg	Sodium <2,300 mg	Carbs grams	Fiber grams	Food Group
Totals								

Depression

Target

Your target is ***to control or relieve symptoms of depression.***

Symptoms of Depression

- Persistent depressed, sad, anxious, or empty mood.
- Feeling worthless, helpless, or guilty.
- Feeling hopeless about the future.
- Losing interest or pleasure in usual activities.
- Chronic fatigue.
- Faulty memory, difficulty concentrating or making decisions.
- Increased irritability, restlessness, or agitation.
- Sleeping either too much or too little.
- Loss of appetite or a tendency to overeat.
- Recurring thoughts of death or suicide.

How to Help Yourself

The following expert advice is offered by the National Institutes of Health (NIH Publication No. 00-3561) on how to help yourself if you are depressed.

- Set realistic goals in light of the depression and assume a reasonable amount of responsibility.
- Break large tasks into small ones, set some priorities, and do what you can as you are able.
- Try to be with other people and to confide in someone; it is usually better than being alone and secretive.
- Participate in activities that may make you feel better.
- Mild exercise, going to a movie or a ball game, or participating in religious, social, or other activities may help.
- Expect your mood to improve gradually, not immediately. Feeling better takes time.
- Try to postpone important decisions until your depression has lifted. Before deciding to make a significant transition—change jobs, get married, or get divorced—discuss it with others who know you well

and have a more objective view of your situation.

- People rarely snap out of a depression. But they can feel a little better day by day.
- *Remember*, positive thinking will replace the negative thinking that is part of the depression and that will disappear as your depression responds to treatment.
- Let your family and friends help you.

How to Help a Family Member or Friend

The most important thing anyone can do for a depressed person is to help him or her get an appropriate diagnosis and treatment.

- Encourage the person to stay with treatment until symptoms begin to abate (this usually takes at least several weeks), or to seek different treatment if there is no improvement.
- If necessary, schedule an appointment and accompany the person to the healthcare provider.
- Monitor whether the person is taking his or her medication.
- Encourage the person to follow the provider's instructions about the use of alcohol while taking medication.
- Offer emotional support: understanding, patience, affection, and encouragement.
- Engage the person in conversation and listen carefully.
- Do not criticize feelings expressed, but point out realities and offer hope.
- Do not ignore remarks about suicide. Report them to the person's healthcare provider.
- Invite the person for walks, outings, movies, and other activities. Be gently insistent if your invitation is refused.
- Encourage participation in some activities that once gave the depressed person pleasure, such as hobbies, sports, and religious or cultural activities, but do not push the person to undertake too much too soon. The person needs diversion and company, but too many demands can increase feelings of failure.
- Do not accuse the person of faking illness or of laziness, or expect him or her "to snap out of it."

- Keep reassuring the person that, with time and help, he or she will feel better.

Therapies for Depression

Your relationship with your healthcare provider is very important. You need to be partners in treating your depression. There are a variety of effective therapies, any or all of which may be effective for you so long as your relationship with your provider is trusting and strong.

- **Talking therapies** help you gain insight into and resolve your problems through verbal exchange with the therapist, sometimes combined with homework assignments between sessions.
- **Behavioral therapies** help you learn how to obtain more satisfaction and rewards through your own actions and how to unlearn the behavioral patterns that contribute to or result from your depression.
- **Interpersonal therapies** focus on your disturbed personal relationships that both cause and exacerbate the depression.
- **Cognitive / behavioral therapies** help you change the negative styles of thinking and behaving often associated with depression.
- **Group therapies and support groups** can help reverse the isolation you may feel and give you the opportunity to be with others suffering similar problems.
- **Electroconvulsive therapy (ECT)** is generally reserved for people whose depression is severe or life-threatening. The procedure is done under anesthesia and with the use of muscle relaxants. Electrodes are placed on the head, and electrical impulses are used to provoke a seizure that lasts about 30 seconds. Usually, several sessions of ECT are required. This therapy can be dramatically effective for major depression, and many people have improved with it. However, side effects including memory loss and impaired thinking can occur in some people as a result of the treatments.

Medications for Depression

As of this writing, most current anti-depressant medications act on the neurotransmitters described in the chapter on depression risk. Anti-depressants are *not* addictive. They must be taken for at least 4 weeks before it can be determined whether or not they are helping you. They are most effective when continued for at least a year or two.

The medications listed below are given as brand name (starting with a capital letter) followed by a generic name (all in small letters).

- **Selective serotonin reuptake inhibitors (SSRIs):** Drugs in this group include *Zoloft / sertraline, Prozac / fluoxetine, Paxil / paroxetine, Celexa / citalopram, Lexapro / escitalopram, Effexor / venlafaxine*, and *Cymbalta / duloxetine.* These boost levels of both norepinephrine and serotonin. SSRIs are the most commonly used class of anti-depressant drugs. (They are also used to treat anxiety disorders.) They work by allowing your body to build up its level of serotonin (a neurotransmitter) plus make better use of the serotonin your body has. The drugs work by inhibiting the uptake of serotonin back into the neurons, by blocking it at the synapse. The result is an improvement of some forms of anxiety disorders and depression.
- **Norepinephrine and dopamine reuptake inhibitors (NDRIs):** An example of a drug in this group is *Wellbutrin / bupropion*. This drug is used for people who do not respond to SSRIs or who experience a slowing in their thought processes or are too sleepy while taking SSRIs. (This same drug, under another name, Zyban, is also used together with nicotine replacement to help people quit smoking.)
- **Serotonin and norepinephrine reuptake inhibitors (SNRIs):** Drugs in this group include *Effexor / venlafaxine* and *Cymbalta / duloxetine.* These are also listed with the SSRIs because they are similar. They boost levels of both norepinephrine and serotonin.
- **Serotonin antagonist reuptake inhibitors (SARIs):** Drugs in this group include *Serzone / nefazodone* and *Desyrel / trazodone.* These work by blocking serotonin from attaching to the receiving nerve or neuroreceptor. This results in an increase in the level of serotonin in the synapse.
- **Tricyclic anti-depressants (TCAs):** Drugs in this group *include Elavil / amitriptyline, Sinequan / doxepin,* and *Tofranil / imipramine.* TCAs are the oldest anti-depressants used today. They, like the SSRIs, work by raising the levels of neurotransmitters in your brain. The SSRIs are used more frequently, but some people benefit from TCAs. Certain

people should not take TCAs because of possible side effects; these include people who have had a recent heart attack, have serious liver disease, are pregnant or breast-feeding, and / or drink alcohol excessively. Your healthcare provider will advise you if this medication is recommended for you.

- **Monoamine oxidase inhibitors (MAOIs):** Drugs in this group include *Marplan / isocarboxazid, Nardil / phenelzine,* and *Parnate / tranylcypromine*. MAOIs are usually reserved for people who do not respond to other treatments. That is because there is a risk of severe hypertension (called *hypertensive crisis*) if you do not follow certain dietary restrictions. Also, these drugs have interactions with many other drugs.

Medications for Bipolar Disorder

Some people experience depression as part of bipolar disorder. The medications used to treat bipolar disorder differ somewhat from the medications used to treat regular depression. Note: Women of childbearing age must be very careful because bipolar medications can have harmful effects on unborn and nursing infants.

- **Lithium:** This medication has mood-stabilizing effects. Because it acts at a certain blood level in your body, you must have blood tests to monitor your level. Often other medications are used with lithium. By working with your mental health professional, you can find the best possible combination.
- **Anti-convulsants:** Drugs in this group include *Tegretol / carbamazepine, Depakote / valproic acid, Lamictal / lamotrigine, Neurontin / gabapentin,* and *Topamax / topiramate.* Anti-convulsants are used with lithium, on their own, or in combination with each other. These medications also have mood-stabilizing effects.

It usually takes bipolar medications four to eight weeks to control your symptoms. You typically keep taking them for six months to one year after an episode of major depression to prevent a relapse. For depressions that continue to recur and for bipolar disorder, you may need to take medications for the rest of your life.

Alternative Medications

> *Special Note: Do not take alternative medications without discussing them first with your healthcare provider.*

They may interact with other medications you are taking. You should not take alternative medications without your healthcare provider's advice if you are taking any of the anti-depressant medications listed above.

- **St. John's wort:** This is a perennial flowering plant whose scientific name is *Hypericum perforatum*. It has been used medicinally for thousands of years. It has been shown in clinical trials to be effective for treating mild and moderate depression. Its mechanism is similar to that of the SSRIs. The standard dose is 300 mg taken three times a day. No studies have been done examining its long-term effects. Don't use it if you are already taking a standard anti-depressant unless you consult your provider. Your provider should be informed if you are taking it in order to note this in your medical records as well as review possible interactions with other medications you may be taking. St. John's wort is officially classified as a dietary supplement. It is not regulated.
- **SAMe:** SAMe is short for *S-adenosylmethionine*. This is not an herbal remedy like St. John's wort, but a natural substance produced by your liver to help various functions in your body. Its mechanism of action is not clearly understood, but it is believed to affect your brain chemistry in a similar way to the SSRIs. In addition to its anti-depressant and anti-anxiety effects, it also appears to function as an anti-inflammatory and helps ease arthritis pain. Also, some studies indicate it may help normalize liver function in people with cirrhosis, hepatitis, and cholestasis (blockage of the bile ducts). The dose is 400 to 1,600 mg per day. Because SAMe is absorbed mainly through your intestine, it is best taken in enteric-coated tablets that pass through your stomach intact. It is advised to start at a low dose (400 mg) taken twice a day on an empty stomach then gradually increase the dose as needed. It is important that you get enough B vitamins, too. Because no studies have been done examining its long-term effects, consult your healthcare provider before taking SAMe. That way, your

provider knows and can note this in your medical records. He or she can also review possible interactions with other medication you may be taking. SAMe is officially classified as a dietary supplement. It is not regulated.

Resources

National Institute of Mental Health (NIMH)
Public Information and Communications Branch
6001 Executive Boulevard, Room 8184, MSC 9663
Bethesda, MD 20892
1-866-615-6464
http://www.nimh.nih.gov/

National Mental Health Association
2000 N. Beauregard Street, 6th Floor
Alexandria, VA 22311
1-800-969-NMHA (6642)
http://www.nmha.org/

American Psychological Association
750 First Street NE
Washington, DC 20002-4242
1-800-374-2721
http://www.apa.org

Stress and Anxiety

Target

No one can tell you whether the stress and anxiety levels in your life are where they should be—only you know the answer to that. However, if you can answer *yes* to the questions posed in the table below, you have the basic coping mechanisms needed to deal with stress and anxiety in your life.

Stress and Anxiety Coping Tools / Targets

I possess the skills I need to handle my stress or anxiety.	❑ Yes	❑ No
I have support and help available when I need it.	❑ Yes	❑ No
I feel safe or can find safety when I need it.	❑ Yes	❑ No
I believe in my power to influence my life circumstances.	❑ Yes	❑ No

Life has a way of stressing us in the exact way that challenges us most. Dancers rarely break fingers and piano players rarely break toes. So every healthy individual should have a tool chest of coping skills to deal with both the predictable and unpredictable curves life throws at them.

The following are methods and techniques you can use to reduce your stress and anxiety.

- **Relaxation techniques:** These are methods of quieting your mind and body. They are easy to learn and get better with practice. Meditation, biofeedback, and progressive relaxation have been proved to slow the heart rate, lower blood pressure, slow respiration, and enhance feelings of well-being. (See Dr. Herbert Benson's book, *The Relaxation Response,* for more on this method.)
- **Cognitive restructuring:** This is a method of choosing positive and powerful thoughts over negative and helpless ones. In other words, you reframe how you look at circumstances. Cognitive therapy is a type of psychotherapy used by mental health professionals to treat anxiety disorders and depression.

- **Exercise:** Exercise is one of the best stress reducers there is, and it comes with a long list of other benefits, too.
- **Eating a well-balanced diet:** Eating a diet that is balanced and includes foods high in nutrients and without excess caffeine, alcohol, sugar, or other stimulants helps control mood, stress, and anxiety.
- **Adequate sleep:** Getting enough sleep is a powerful weapon against stress. Americans are notoriously sleep-deprived. Without adequate sleep and rest, you more quickly reach a point of exhaustion, where your energy to repel stress is overwhelmed.
- **Recreation and time for unstructured play:** These will reduce stress and anxiety and provide insights into how to best handle the stressors in your life. Children play to practice skills they will need later in life; that's why play is a child's job. As adults, we often miss out on discovering our happiest strengths (strengths that will help us repel stress) because we don't allow ourselves time to simply play at things that amuse us.
- **Social support:** Support from others is essential to prevent feelings of isolation and loneliness. Nothing is more reassuring when you are stressed than talking your concern over with a trusted friend, family member, or healthcare provider. Misery really does love company, and knowing others understand what you are going through makes everything easier.
- **Spiritual meaning in your life:** This comfort will carry you through all of life's adversity. It is a well from which you can drink over and over and always be refreshed. In times of stress and anxiety, go often to your place of spiritual peace, whether it is a place inside yourself or an outside house of worship.

Therapy for Stress and Anxiety

If you suffer everyday stress and aren't happy with the role it plays in your life, using the strategies outlined in this Appendix and the chapter on mental resilience (Your Third Choice: *Mental Resilience*) can help you take control of the stress in your life. If you have an anxiety disorder, you may need the help of a mental health professional who will use a combination of psychotherapy and medication to help you bring your anxiety disorder under control.

Cognitive-behavioral therapy is a method of treatment in which you engage in a dialogue with a trained therapist for the purpose of helping you understand the nature of your anxiety. You and your therapist focus on the here and now (versus psychotherapy, where you delve into your past). A goal-directed, problem-solving approach is used to help you decrease or eliminate your anxiety reactions. This kind of therapy is usually a time-limited treatment lasting anywhere from 4 to 16 weeks. During this therapy, you are given homework assignments to complete on your own and bring to your next session. You also are encouraged to take responsibility for certain aspects of your problem. You are helped to discover behaviors that will decrease your anxiety and to learn to express your feelings appropriately.

Medication for Stress and Anxiety

Four classes of medications are used to treat anxiety disorders. The particular one that is right for you must be chosen carefully by your healthcare provider. It is important that you completely understand its effects and side effects. Tell your provider about any alternative therapies or over-the-counter medications you are using. Ask when and how the medication will be stopped. Some drugs should not be stopped abruptly; they have to be tapered down slowly, under your provider's supervision. Be aware that some medications are effective for treating anxiety disorders only as long as they are taken regularly; that is, your symptoms may recur when the medications are stopped. Work with your provider to determine the right dose of the right medication to treat your anxiety disorder.

The following are the classes of medicine used to treat anxiety. They are listed with their brand name first (starting with a capital letter) and their generic name second (in all small letters).

- **Selective serotonin reuptake inhibitors (SSRIs):** Drugs in this group include *Zoloft / sertraline, Prozac / fluoxetine, Paxil / paroxetine, Celexa / citalopram, Lexapro / escitalopram, Effexor / venlafaxine,* and *Cymbalta / duloxetine.* SSRIs are the most commonly used class of anti-depressant drugs and are also used to treat anxiety disorders. They work by maintaining normal levels of certain chemicals in your brain called neurotransmitters. This improves some forms of both anxiety disorders and depression. SSRIs are not addictive. They must be taken for at least 4 weeks before you will know if they are helping. They are most effective when continued for at least a year or two.

- **Tricyclic anti-depressants (TCAs):** Drugs in this group include *Elavil / amitriptyline, Sinequan / doxepin,* and *Tofranil / imipramine*. TCAs are the oldest anti-depressants we use today. They, like SSRIs, work by raising the levels of neurotransmitters in your brain. The SSRIs are used more frequently, but some people benefit from TCAs. Certain people should not take TCAs because of possible side effects; these include people who have had a recent heart attack, have serious liver disease, are pregnant or breast-feeding, and / or drink alcohol excessively. Your healthcare provider will advise you if this medication is recommended for you.
- **Benzodiazepines:** Drugs in this group include *Xanax / alprazolam, Klonopin / clonazepam, Ativan / lorazepam,* and *Valium / diazepam*. Benzodiazepines were first developed in the 1960s. They control anxiety. They work by binding to certain receptors in your brain called *GABA receptors*. The binding results in sedation and a sense of tranquility. These drugs are addictive, so they are not recommended for long-term or continuous use. They also are not recommended for people who have a history of substance abuse. Taken in combination with alcohol, they can be toxic, even deadly.
- **Non-benzodiazepine anxiolytics:** Drugs in this group include *BuSpar / buspirone* and *Vistaril / hydroxyzine*. These are a class of drugs used for anxiety that work in a variety of different ways. Because drugs from this class are not addictive, they are safer to use than benzodiazepines if you have a history of substance abuse.

Alternative Medications

Special Note: Do not take alternative medications without discussing them first with your healthcare provider. They may interact with other medications you are taking. You should not take alternative medications without your healthcare provider's advice if you are taking any of the medications listed above.

- **St. John's wort:** This is a perennial flowering plant whose scientific name is *Hypericum perforatum*. Used medicinally for thousands of years, it has been shown in clinical trials to be effective in treating mild and moderate depression. Its mechanism is similar to that of the SSRIs. The standard dose is 300 mg taken three times a day. Don't use it if you are already taking a prescribed anti-depressant unless your healthcare provider advises it. Because no studies have been done examining St. John's wort's long-term effects, consult your provider before taking it. It should be noted that you are taking it in your medical records, as it may interact with medications you are taking. St. John's wort is officially classified as a dietary supplement. It is not regulated.
- **Kava:** This is an extract from the root of the pepper plant *Piper methysticum*. It comes from the South Pacific, where it has been part of social rituals and traditional medicine for centuries. Kava acts on the emotional center of your brain, producing a sense of tranquility and softening feelings of anger and fear. **Warning: The Food and Drug Administration has advised caution with kava supplements because of a potential risk of severe liver injury, including cirrhosis and liver failure.** Discuss this supplement with your healthcare provider to get the most up-to-date information about its potential dangers. If you take this supplement, do not mix it with alcohol or other drugs that affect your brain, and do not do anything that requires being alert, such as driving. Also, if used for a long time, kava can cause scaling of your skin. An effective daily dose of kava is between 70 and 200 mg of kavalactones. Because no studies have been done examining its long-term effects, consult your provider before taking it. It should be noted you are taking it in your medical records, as it may interact with medications you are taking. Kava is officially classified as a dietary supplement. It is not regulated.
- **SAMe:** SAMe is short for *S-adenosylmethionine*. This is not an herbal remedy like St. John's wort, but a natural substance produced by your liver to help various functions in your body. Its mechanism of action is not clearly understood, but it is believed to affect your brain

chemistry in a similar way to the SSRIs. In addition to its anti-depressant and anti-anxiety effects, it also appears to function as an anti-inflammatory and help ease arthritis pain. Some studies indicate it may help normalize liver function in people with cirrhosis, hepatitis, and cholestasis (blockage of the bile ducts). The dose is 400 to 1,600 mg per day. Because SAMe is absorbed mainly through your intestine, it is best taken in enteric-coated tablets that pass through your stomach intact. It is advised to start at a low dose (400 mg) taken twice a day on an empty stomach and to gradually increase the dose as needed. It is important that you get enough B vitamins, too. Because no studies have been done examining SAMe's long-term effects, consult your healthcare provider before taking it. It should be noted you are taking it in your medical records, as it may interact with medications you are taking. SAMe is officially classified as a dietary supplement. It is not regulated.

Resources

Anxiety Disorders Association of America (ADAA)
8730 Georgia Avenue, Suite 600
Silver Spring, MD 20910
1-240-485-1001
http://www.adaa.org

National Mental Health Association
2000 N. Beauregard Street, 6th Floor
Alexandria, VA 22311
1-800-969-NMHA (6642)
http://www.nmha.org/

National Institute of Mental Health (NIMH)
Public Information and Communications Branch
6001 Executive Boulevard, Room 8184, MSC 9663
Bethesda, MD 20892
1-866-615-6464
http://www.nimh.nih.gov/

American Psychological Association
750 First Street NE
Washington, DC 20002-4242
1-800-374-2721
http://www.apa.org/

Alcohol

Target

Your target is to drink *no more than* the amount of alcohol that is safe for you. Different parts of the world propose different safe amounts of alcohol consumption for men and women. Moderate alcohol consumption, according to guidelines used in the United States, is the following.

Alcohol Safe Limits per Day

Type of alcohol	Men	Women
Beer	24 oz.	12 oz.
Wine	10 oz.	5 oz.
Hard liquor	1 oz.	½ oz.

U.S. Department of Health Dietary Guidelines for Americans

Women's safe amounts are smaller than men's because of their smaller body size and different metabolisms. In addition, every individual has his or her own unique physical and genetic susceptibilities to alcohol. Health complications such as alcoholism or liver disease may result with any alcohol consumption at all.

If you drink more than recommended amounts of alcohol, you are at risk. The best way to handle this risk, as with any other, is by being aware of the potential danger. Be alert to your drinking behaviors. Be honest with yourself about who is in control—you or the alcohol.

If you already abuse alcohol or have become dependent on alcohol, you will need the help of a medical professional to manage your alcohol problem. Because alcohol is a depressant, people with alcohol problems often have problems with depression or anxiety, too. These can be successfully treated, and you can gain control over not only your alcohol intake, but also your depression and anxiety.

Steps You Can Take

The following are steps you can take on your own to reduce or eliminate your risks from alcohol.

- **Keep a "cocktail diary" for a week.** Write down every drink you have and measure the quantity. Do not freshen drinks without measuring.

Note the date, time of day, what you are drinking, and how you are feeling. Are you drinking more or less than what is considered a safe amount for your gender (see the table above)?

- **Try to identify your drinking cues.** Do you always have a drink after work, when you smoke, with certain foods or meals, in certain places, or with certain people?
- **Write down a drinking goal and make a contract to stick to it.**
- **Buy some self-help books about problem drinking. Attend Alcoholics Anonymous (AA) meetings for group support.**
- **Consider the potential health problems mentioned above.** Do you already suffer from any of them? Are you at risk for alcohol abuse or dependence? Do you suffer from alcohol abuse or dependence? Do you have family members who do?
- **Try to stop drinking or cut back.** Is it a problem for you? Are you in control of the alcohol, or is it in control of you? If it is in control of you, you need to stop drinking *completely*. If you can't do this without physical or psychological symptoms, seek the care of a medical professional.
- **If your drinking is out of control, or you can't stop drinking without having physical or psychological symptoms, do not try to stop on your own—get help.** Alcohol withdrawal can be dangerous, even fatal, and there is medical care available to help you. Delirium tremens (DTs) is a serious medical condition caused by alcohol withdrawal that can lead to hallucinations, fever, and violence. Alcohol withdrawal seizures are not uncommon in people who suddenly stop heavy drinking. Call 911 and go to the nearest emergency room if you need help.
- **Remain optimistic and hopeful.** Cessation of alcohol will lead to greater happiness, increased self-respect, and improved physical and emotional health.

Your first 12 weeks are critical to staying sober for the long term.

Healthcare providers use medications to wean you off the alcohol. This is called *detoxification* or *detox*. After detoxification, other medications help you maintain your abstinence from alcohol. Medications used for alcohol detoxification reverse the symptoms of alcohol withdrawal.

Medications to Treat Alcohol Withdrawal

The most common medications used to treat alcohol withdrawal symptoms are *benzodiazepines* (given with their Brand Name / generic name): *Ativan / lorazepam, Valium / diazepam,* and *Librium / chlordiazepoxide.* These can be given intravenously (IV), orally, or by injection. They are carefully tapered off as your body adjusts to being without alcohol. The medications prevent seizures and help you feel more comfortable as you come off the alcohol.

People who abuse alcohol are vitamin-depleted, so during alcohol detoxification, the following supplements are given:

- Thiamine
- Folic acid
- Magnesium
- Multivitamins

Medications to Help You Stay Sober

The following medications are used in helping maintain sobriety.

- ***Antabuse / disulfiram:*** This drug interferes with alcohol metabolism. As a result, you become very uncomfortable and nauseated if you consume alcohol.
- ***ReVia / naltrexone:*** This drug decreases your urge to drink. People who relapse while taking naltrexone drink less alcohol and have less severe relapses than those not taking this drug.
- **Selective serotonin reuptake inhibitors (SSRIs):** Drugs in this group include *Zoloft / sertraline, Prozac / fluoxetine, Paxil / paroxetine, Effexor / venlafaxine,* and *Celexa / citalopram.* The SSRIs are a class of anti-depressant drugs that are also used for the treatment of alcohol problems.

Resources

National Clearinghouse for Alcohol and Drug Information (NCADI)
11420 Rockville Pike
Rockville, MD 20852
1-800-729-6686 (24 hours a day, 7 days a week)
http://ncadi.samhsa.gov/

Alcoholics Anonymous World Services, Inc.
P.O. Box 459
New York, NY 10163
1-212- 870-3400
http://www.alcoholics-anonymous.org

Smoking

Target

If you smoke, your target is to quit. Quitting tobacco is *hard*. Experts say it is harder to stop smoking than it is to get off heroin or cocaine. Most people try to quit *two or three times* before they are permanently successful. In spite of that, according to the Surgeon General, 46 million Americans have successfully quit for good. Most of them agree that life really is better without tobacco.

Smoking Target :
Complete Cessation of Tobacco Use

Get Ready, Get Set, Quit

- The first step to quitting smoking is to imagine yourself as a non-smoker. Imagine all the ways your life will be better without cigarettes. Make a list of all the reasons you want to quit, and keep it handy for later when you have cravings.
- Next, prepare yourself mentally. Get psyched up. Know you are getting ready to do something big, brave, and hard. Prepare to do battle against your addiction to cigarettes or whatever tobacco product you use. Create images in your mind . . . see yourself overcoming temptations, choosing over and over again not to smoke, and having better things to do besides smoking.
- Set a quit date, ideally within the next two weeks.
- See your healthcare provider for medication, nicotine replacement, and / or counseling before your quit date.
- Sign up with a program or a telephone quit line to give you support. Planning ahead will increase your chances of success.
- Tell your family, friends, and co-workers about your plan to quit and ask for their support and understanding.
- Make a battle plan—it will be a battle and you want to be *ready*. Think of healthy ways to deal with withdrawal symptoms and cravings. Gum, toothpicks, hard candies, or lozenges can help keep your mouth busy without adding too many calories.

- Discover your smoking triggers and avoid them if you can. For example, if you always have a cigarette with coffee in the morning, switch to tea instead.
- In the two weeks before quitting, avoid smoking in places where you spend a lot of time—home, work, the car, etc. This helps you get used to being in familiar environments without cigarettes and will decrease their effect of triggering you to light up.
- Stay out of places where smokers tend to congregate, like bars.
- Avoid alcohol for several weeks—it lowers your defenses and may cause you to impulsively light up.
- Drink lots and lots of water, particularly at first. It will flush the nicotine and toxins out of your body. You may also find that water, fruits, vegetables, and salads are appealing in ways they never were when you were smoking. Enjoy them all you want. They won't cause you to gain weight.
- Exercise is a wonderful antidote to nicotine cravings. Get out in the open air and breathe. Walking or running will control weight gain, improve fitness, and give you a mental boost.
- Remove all tobacco products (cigarettes, ashtrays, lighters, etc.) from your environment. When they are out of the house or office and you have cravings, you will be reminded of your resolve and commitment.
- Go to the dentist on or after your quit day to get your teeth cleaned.
- Clean and air out your house, car, and clothing (including closets).

Medications for Smoking Cessation

- ***Chantix / varenicline tartrate:*** This is the newest drug for smoking cessation approved by the Food and Drug Administration in May of 2006. Just like bupropion, you take it for 12 to 24 weeks. It acts on nicotine receptors in your brain and helps you quit in two ways: it decreases your cravings for nicotine and reduces your urge to smoke.
- ***Zyban and Wellbutrin / bupropion:*** This is an anti-depressant drug that is effective in helping with smoking cessation either with or without nicotine replacement. You take it for 12 to 24 weeks. You must have a prescription from your healthcare provider. You should not take it if you have ever had a seizure.

- **Nicotine replacement:** You can purchase nicotine replacement over the counter without a prescription. It comes in patches, gum, lozenges, and inhalants. The patches come in three strengths and are gradually tapered down over 12 to 16 weeks. The gum is chewed only as needed to suppress cravings. Do not use nicotine replacement while you are still smoking because you could suffer nicotine overdose. If you have coronary artery disease, see your healthcare provider before starting nicotine replacement. If you are taking Chantix, you shouldn't need nicotine replacement.

Support for Smoking Cessation

- **Smoking cessation intensive group therapy:** This is a kind of program usually run by your local hospital or the Red Cross. This therapy can be very effective: It helps to go through the process of quitting with others who are in the same boat.
- **American Cancer Society Quit Lines:** These quit lines are phone-counseling programs that have been shown to double the chances of quitting permanently. These programs are getting started in many states. Check with your local health department or the American Cancer Society to see if there is a Quit Line in your community. Note: This program can be combined with Chantix, Zyban, or nicotine replacement.

Resources

U.S. Department of Health and Human Services
Office of the Surgeon General
600 Fishers Lane
Room 18-66
Rockville, MD 20857
1-301-443-4000
http://www.surgeongeneral.gov/tobacco/

Cancer

Cancer Screening Tests

Screening tests are done to check for cancer when you *do not have any symptoms*. Some screenings are examinations that you do yourself (like self–breast exams, self–testicular exams, or notifying your healthcare provider if you notice that a mole or wart is changing). Other screenings (like a PAP smear and prostate exam) are part of your routine physical examinations. Also, some screenings are performed by someone other than your regular healthcare provider. For example, a mammogram is done at an x-ray center, and a colonoscopy is performed by a medical specialist called a gastroenterologist.

The American Cancer Society recommends the following cancer screenings.

Breast Cancer	Women should perform self–breast exams and have clinical breast exams (that is, ones performed by their healthcare providers), and a yearly mammogram starting at age 40 and continuing as long as a woman is in good health. Screenings are started earlier in women who have a history of breast cancer in their family.
Cervical Cancer	Screening PAP smears should begin within 3 years after a woman begins having vaginal intercourse and no later than age 21. PAPs should be done every year. After age 30, women who have had three normal PAPs in a row may be screened every 2 to 3 years unless they are at high risk (talk to your provider about your cervical cancer risks). After a total hysterectomy, PAP smears may be discontinued *unless* cervical cancer was the reason for the hysterectomy. Women over the age of 70 may stop having PAP smears if they have had three or more normal smears in the prior 10 years.

Colon and Rectal Cancer	You should have a fecal occult blood test every year starting at age 50 and a screening colonoscopy every 5 to 10 years based on the recommendation of the gastroenterologist who performs it.
Oral Cancer	You should have an examination of your mouth by a medical or dental health professional.
Prostate Cancer	Men should have a digital rectal exam *and* a PSA (prostate-specific antigen) blood test every year starting at age 50 and continuing as long as their life expectancy is greater than 10 years. Men at high risk (African Americans and men who have had a relative who got prostate cancer at a young age) should start screenings at age 45.
Skin Cancer	You should have a skin survey. This is an examination in which the skin on your entire body is examined under good light and magnification to look for suspicious lesions. Biopsies (collection of a small sample of tissue) are performed as needed.
Testicular Cancer	Men should perform self–testicular exams and have a clinical exam performed at their routine physical examination.

Cancer Testing

Because each type of cancer is unique, each requires specialized diagnostic testing. Covering all these possible tests is beyond the scope of this book. Certain tests are used frequently in medicine for diagnosing a wide variety of diseases—including cancer—and those tests are discussed below.

In diagnosing and treating cancer, some testing is done to find out *if you have a cancer* and some testing is done to see *how far the cancer has spread once it has been discovered.* Testing to see how far a cancer has spread is called *staging* and is described in more detail later in this section. The following tests are used commonly in the diagnosis and staging of many types of cancers.

- **Biopsy and cytology tests:** These are tests in which tissue or cells are taken from your body and examined under a microscope by a medical specialist called a pathologist. These tests directly identify cancer cells and can determine their exact type. A PAP smear is an example of a cytology test. Cells are scraped from a woman's cervix and examined under a microscope to see if they are abnormal or cancerous. Some biopsies may be done using local anesthesia in an office. This means you are given anesthesia that numbs just one part of your body and you stay awake. For example, skin biopsies are usually performed in your healthcare provider's office. Other biopsies may be performed in an operating room with you completely asleep under general anesthesia. This is done when the tissue sample is difficult to reach, as in lung biopsies, for example.

- **Ultrasound:** This test is also called sonography. It uses a metal bulb as a sensor that is rubbed across your skin after a gel has been applied. The ultrasound machine creates images from the sound waves and shows them on a monitor screen. An ultrasound is not painful. It can show whether a mass or lump is filled with fluid or is solid. Ultrasound is often used to guide needle biopsies to the right place.
- **Endoscopy:** During endoscopy, a flexible scope—a tube with a tiny camera on the end—is inserted into a part of the body. By using this test, your healthcare provider can not only see inside your body (and put what he or she sees on a monitor for you to see as well), but also take tissue samples. A colonoscopy is an example of an endoscopy test that looks for cancer in the colon and is able to remove precancerous polyps (or growths) that are seen during the test. Endoscopy can be used in many places in your body, such as your throat, lungs, esophagus, stomach, abdominal cavity, uterus, and bladder. You are sedated for this test.
- **X-rays:** These are also called radiographs. They use radiation that is beamed through your body and casts shadows onto film. The film is read by specialists called radiologists. X-rays are used to detect tumors. Mammograms are examples of x-rays used to screen for and diagnose breast cancer. Sometimes x-rays are done with a substance called contrast. This is given either orally or through an intravenous

line (IV) and causes certain structures in your body to light up, making them easier to see. X-rays are painless. You get a small amount of radiation from them, but this is not usually enough to be dangerous if you do not have repeated exposure to higher radiation levels than are used in most diagnostic x-rays. Newer tests like CT scans and MRI scans (described below) have replaced x-rays in many situations, but x-rays are still commonly used diagnostic tools.

- **CT scan:** This scan is also called a CAT scan. It stands for computed (axial) tomography. This test uses a computer and looks at your body in slices. Imagine lying on the table and having your body viewed in paper-thin slices, from the top of your head to the bottoms of your feet. That's how a CT scan looks at you. This scan uses radiation, like x-rays, but the radiation is a thin beam that the computer then constructs into images the radiologist can read. CT scans are used for many purposes, including identifying the shape, size, and location of a tumor. This scan can also reveal any blood vessels that are feeding a tumor. It can help guide a needle biopsy to a tumor, measure a cancer's shrinkage after treatment with radiation or chemotherapy, and detect if a cancer has recurred. Sometimes this test is done with a substance called contrast. This is given either orally or through an intravenous line (IV) and causes certain structures in your body to light up on the scan, making them easier to see. Like x-rays, this test is not painful. The CT scan is used in detecting and evaluating cancer in your liver, pancreas, adrenal glands, lungs, and bones. It is also used to provide information about cancer in your large and small intestines, esophagus, stomach, or brain. The CT scan can help assess the stage of prostate cancer, too.
- **Spiral CT scan:** The spiral CT scan is a painless procedure in which a special CT machine rotates rapidly around your body, taking more than 100 pictures in sequence. The scan is so sensitive that it can detect nodules that are too small to be seen on a regular x-ray. Low-radiation spiral CT scans are emerging as one of the most promising tools in the early detection of lung cancer. The National Cancer Institute does not yet accept this scan as a screening tool for lung

cancer, but as of this writing, these scans are being studied in clinical trials. If you're at risk for lung cancer, talk with your healthcare provider about enrolling in one of these trials. Currently, most medical insurance will not pay for general lung cancer screening using the low-radiation spiral CT scan, and the tests are very expensive.

- **MRI scan:** MRI stands for magnetic resonant imaging. Instead of using radiation, it uses a powerful magnet and radio waves to create very detailed images of the structures inside your body. Because it uses a strong magnet, you must remove all metal from the outside of your body before the test. Some people, like those with metal inside their bodies from previous surgeries, cannot have MRIs. Be sure to tell your healthcare provider if you have any metal in your body. This includes pacemakers, surgical clips, or older stents from coronary angioplasty. Having an MRI scan feels like being in a tunnel, and this makes some people nervous. If you have claustrophobia, tell your healthcare provider before the test. There are both open and closed MRIs. If you have claustrophobia, your provider may schedule you for an open MRI, which does not have the enclosed space. An MRI scan is not painful, but the machine makes a loud banging noise when it is operating; you are given headphones so the technician can talk to you during the procedure and you can listen to music. The test takes a long time (usually 45 minutes to 2 hours) during which you need to lie very still. Sometimes this test is done using a substance called contrast. This is given either orally or through an intravenous line (IV) and causes certain structures in your body to light up on the scan, making them easier to see. The MRI scan is best at detecting cancer in your brain and spinal cord, head, neck, female reproductive tract, and musculoskeletal system. It is also used to look for signs that cancer has metastasized to your liver from another part of your body.
- **Nuclear scans:** These are also called radionuclide imaging. In nuclear scans (unlike other types of tests with contrast), the type of contrast used has a very small amount of radiation, called tracers, that you swallow or that are injected into your bloodstream. Tissues affected by cancer may absorb more or less of the tracer than normal tissues.

A special camera photographs where the tracers have gone and detects hot spots and cold spots. Hot spots are where more of the tracer has been absorbed; cold spots are where less of the tracer has been absorbed. A cancer may show up as either a hot spot or a cold spot, but either way, it stands out as different from the surrounding normal tissue. The radiation used in this scan is about the same as that used for a regular x-ray. Nuclear scans are used to locate tumors, especially in your bones and thyroid. They are also used to tell the stage once a cancer has been discovered and to determine if a treatment is working. Nuclear scans may detect very small tumors, but they will not distinguish between benign and malignant tumors. A PET scan is one type of nuclear scan; this scan can detect the metabolic activity of a tumor (how quickly it is growing) as well as its location and size.

Cancer Staging

Different types of cancer can cause virtually any type of symptom. As a cancer progresses, it goes through stages, producing more symptoms as it goes. The symptoms will depend on the size of the cancer, its location, its effect on the surrounding organs or structures, and whether it has metastasized. *Staging* is the process of finding out if the cancer has spread and, if so, by how much. The following is from the American Cancer Society and describes the process of staging.

A cancer's stage is based on information about the original (primary) tumor:

- The tumor's size.
- Whether or not the tumor has grown into other nearby areas.
- Whether or not the cancer has spread to the surrounding lymph nodes.
- Whether or not the cancer has metastasized (spread) to distant areas of your body.

The ***TNM system*** is the staging system healthcare providers use most. It gives three key pieces of information:

- **T** describes the size of the *tumor*, and whether the cancer has spread to nearby tissues and organs.

- **N** describes how far the cancer has spread to nearby lymph *nodes.*
- **M** shows whether the cancer has *metastasized* (spread) to other organs of your body.

Letters or numbers after the T, N, and M give more details about each of these factors. For example, a cancer classified as *T1, N0, M0* is a tumor that is very small, has not spread to the lymph nodes, and has not spread to distant organs of the body. In general, the *lower* the number, such as stage I, the *less* the cancer has spread. A higher number, such as stage IV, means a more serious, widespread cancer.

Cancer Treatments

The treatment or combination of treatments that is best for any individual with cancer depends on a number of factors. The type of cancer being treated, how advanced it is when it is diagnosed, and the person's age, physical condition, and personal preferences all go into making recommendations about which treatments are best.

The treatment of cancer is highly specific and complex, and far beyond the scope of this book. However, explanations of the four main types of treatment are given below.

For more information, your local library and websites of the American Cancer Society and the National Cancer Institute have extensive and detailed information about individual cancer treatments. Links to these websites and others are included in the resources given at the end of this section.

- **Surgery:** This is the oldest form of cancer treatment. It is recommended when a cancer is contained, has not spread, and can be removed totally to cure the cancer. For example, cervical cancer is completely curable in its early stages by surgically removing the cancerous cells from the cervix or by completely removing the cervix via a hysterectomy. Sometimes surgery is recommended—even if the cancer has metastasized—to help control a person's symptoms (so that he or she has a better quality of life) or to slow the spread of the cancer.
- **Radiation therapy:** This is the use of energy waves in the form of gamma or x-rays (called *ionizing radiation*) to penetrate into the body and interrupt the growth process of cells that are rapidly dividing.

The side effects of radiation therapy occur because the radiation affects nearby normal cells as well as cancerous cells. Radiation is considered a local treatment since only the cells that are radiated are affected by the treatments. Radiation is sometimes used to stop or slow cancer cells from multiplying, thereby slowing the spread of cancer. Lung cancer is one type of cancer that is commonly treated with radiation. Radiation therapy is often used in conjunction with chemotherapy.

- **Chemotherapy:** Having chemotherapy ("chemo") means taking medications that fight cancer. Chemotherapy and radiation therapy are often used together to treat cancer. Medications to treat cancer target cells that grow rapidly—both cancer cells and healthy cells. The *side effects* of chemotherapy come from the drugs' effects on healthy, rapidly growing cells like hair cells (leading to hair loss), stomach cells (leading to nausea), bone marrow cells (leading to anemia and fatigue), and cells in the mouth (leading to mouth sores). These side effects go away after you finish chemotherapy. Chemotherapy is given in many ways: by mouth in pill form, by occasional injections, or through an intravenous line (IV) directly into a vein. You may take chemotherapy once a day, once a week, or once a month: It depends on the type of cancer and the kind of chemotherapy. How long chemotherapy is continued also depends on the type of cancer and what length of chemotherapy research has shown is most effective. New types of chemotherapy are being developed that affect only the cancer cells and leave healthy cells alone.
- **Immunotherapy:** This is a treatment aimed at stimulating your body's own immune system to fight cancer or the side effects of its treatments. It is also called *biologic therapy*. It is currently used along with other therapies, instead of all by itself. Immunotherapy is the newest form of cancer treatment and will become even more promising as scientists figure out new ways of targeting only the cancer cells and leaving healthy cells alone. That is the treatment dream of the future . . . and immunotherapy is a first step toward it. At the present time, surgery, radiation therapy, and chemotherapy

remain the mainstays of cancer treatment. There are many promising treatments for cancer being discovered every day, and treatments continue to get better and better all the time.

Resources

American Cancer Society
1-800-ACS-2345
http://www.cancer.org/docroot/home/index.asp

National Cancer Institute
1-800-4-CANCER
http://www.cancer.gov

National Comprehensive Cancer Network
1-888-909-NCCN
http://www.nccn.gov

Centers for Disease Control and Prevention (CDC)
1-800-CDC-INFO (232-4636)
http://www.cdc.gov/cancer

Glossary of Medical Terms

A

A1c—*see Hemoglobin A1c.*

Angioplasty—an invasive medical procedure in which a wire is threaded into a blood vessel to detect, x-ray, and / or open a blocked or narrowed blood vessel. This procedure can be performed on the blood vessels of your heart (coronary arteries), the main arteries to your kidneys (renal arteries), and / or the vessels of your legs. Sometimes a balloon is attached to the wire and inflated in a blood vessel to expand the vessel and improve blood flow through it. This is called *balloon angioplasty*. Often a small, straw-shaped *stent* is placed in the vessel during the angioplasty to help keep the vessel open.

ARNP—Advanced Registered Nurse Practitioner, *see Nurse Practitioner, NP*

Arteriosclerosis / atherosclerosis—the buildup of fatty substances and plaque composed of different types of cholesterol over your lifetime on the inner walls of your blood vessels. Also called *hardening of the arteries*.

Asthma—an allergic respiratory disorder that causes narrowing of your lung passages, wheezing, and shortness of breath. Degrees of severity can vary from very mild to life-threatening.

B

Biofeedback—a method for learning to control physiologic processes (such as heart rate, blood pressure, muscle tension / relaxation, or stress responses) by using some type of monitoring device that feeds back information on your physiologic state to both you and your healthcare provider.

Blood pressure—a measure of the pressure inside the blood vessels of your body when your heart beats and when your heart rests in between heartbeats. High blood pressure puts stress on all the blood vessels in your body and can lead to heart attack and stroke. Low blood pressure prevents adequate blood flow from reaching your vital organs and can cause dizziness, fainting, or even organ failure.

Body mass index (BMI)—a measure that defines healthy weights based on height. A BMI of 18.5 up to 25 refers to a healthy weight, a BMI of 25 up to 30 refers to overweight, and a BMI of 30 or higher refers to obesity. (See the BMI table and equation in the Weight section in this Appendix.)

BP—*see blood pressure.*

Bronchitis (chronic)—bronchitis is a mucus-producing cough that is present most days of the week and results from inflammation, obstruction, and damage to the air passages (bronchi) of the lungs, usually because of cigarette smoking. Chronic bronchitis is a type of *chronic obstructive pulmonary disease* (COPD).

C

C-reactive protein (CRP)—a plasma protein that rises in response to inflammation; increased levels are believed to increase your risk of cardiovascular disease. If your levels are high, taking 81 mg of aspirin daily (if you are not allergic or have other reasons you should not take aspirin) may reduce risk.

Carcinogen—a substance capable of causing cancer in animals or humans.

Cardiovascular disease—disease of the heart or blood vessels caused by a combination of genetic and lifestyle risk factors.

Carotid arteries—two large blood vessels on either side of your neck that supply blood to your brain.

Carotid artery disease—the buildup of fatty substances and plaque composed of different types of cholesterol in the carotid arteries of your neck that can lead to blockages, plaque rupture, and stroke; a form of *atherosclerosis*.

CBC—complete blood cell count (see "Routine Laboratory Tests" in this Appendix for details).

CHF—*see congestive heart failure.*

Cholestasis—blocked bile duct; can be caused by gallstones, drugs, liver disease, and infection. Sometimes causes jaundice (yellowing of your skin and the whites of your eyes).

Cirrhosis—permanent scarring of your liver that results in its inability to detoxify your blood. May be caused by alcohol abuse, drugs, or infection. Can lead to jaundice (yellowing of your skin and the whites of your eyes), fluid retention, liver failure, and death.

CNA—*see Nurse Assistant, Certified*

Congestive heart failure (CHF)—a condition in which your heart becomes too weak to pump enough blood to keep circulation going; usually caused by a heart attack, uncontrolled blood pressure, or diseases that weaken your heart. Results in a buildup of fluid in your lungs, abdomen, and legs.

COPD—term for two diseases: *chronic bronchitis* and *emphysema*; permanent and irreversible lung damage that gets worse over time; most common cause is smoking. Causes wheezing, difficulty in breathing, and a chronic cough.

Coronary artery disease—the buildup of fatty substances and plaque composed of different types of cholesterol in the arteries that feed your heart (coronary arteries). Can lead to blockages, plaque rupture, and heart attack. A form of *atherosclerosis*.

CVA—Cerebrovascular accident, *see stroke.*

Cytokines—powerful chemical substances secreted by certain cells. These act as chemical messengers. They are involved in both immune and inflammatory responses in your body.

D

DASH diet—**D**ietary **A**pproaches to **S**top **H**ypertension diet; a diet for the treatment of high blood pressure and other diseases such as cancer. The diet is low in sodium (salt) and cholesterol; high in fiber, potassium, calcium, and magnesium; and moderately high in protein.

DBP—*see diastolic blood pressure.*

Delirium tremens (DTs)—a potentially life-threatening condition that results from the sudden cessation of alcohol consumption after a long period of heavy drinking. Characterized by overactivity of your nervous system with shakes, tremors, hallucinations, and seizures.

Detoxification / detox—the process of removing toxins from your body; usually refers to the process of withdrawing from alcohol or other drugs under the supervision of medical professionals.

Diabetic ketoacidosis (DKA)—a medical emergency in which very high blood glucose levels and lack of *insulin* result in the accumulation of ketones in your blood and urine. Occurs because your body breaks down body fat for energy. Nausea, vomiting, stomach pain, fruity breath odor, and rapid breathing are signs of DKA. If untreated, it can lead to coma and death.

Diastolic blood pressure (DBP)—the bottom number in a blood pressure reading; represents the lowest pressure in your blood vessels that occurs when your heart rests in between heartbeats.

Dietary supplement—Congress defined the term *dietary supplement* in the Dietary Supplement Health and Education Act (DSHEA) of 1994 as follows: "A dietary supplement is a product taken by mouth that contains a 'dietary ingredient' intended to supplement the diet." Supplements do not undergo the same clinical testing and approval process that prescription drugs do.

Diuretics / water pills—medications used to treat high blood pressure. They work by increasing urination and promoting the elimination of salt and water by your kidneys. Also used to treat congestive heart failure and some other medical conditions.

DTs—*see delirium tremens.*

E

Echocardiogram—a test that uses sound waves to create a picture of your heart and that can measure the pumping capacity of your heart and the condition of your heart muscle and valves.

Electrocardiogram (ECG, EKG)—a test that records the electrical activity of your heart and can detect rhythm abnormalities and impaired blood flow to your heart as in a heart attack.

Electrolytes—substances in your blood that enable your heart and fluids in your body to work properly. The most important electrolytes are sodium, potassium, and chloride. Abnormal levels can cause heart and other problems. See "Routine Laboratory Tests" for more.

Emphysema—permanent and irreversible damage to your lungs that gets worse over time; most common cause is smoking; symptoms include difficulty in breathing, wheezing, and a chronic cough. *See COPD.*

Endorphins—hormone-like substances produced in your brain that help control pain responses; often called the body's natural morphine.

Enzyme—a protein inside the cells of your body that causes chemical reactions to occur.

F

Fatty liver—an infiltration of fat into the cells of your liver; caused by excess alcohol consumption, diabetes, obesity, and pregnancy. Also called *steatosis*.

G

Gastroparesis—a form of nerve damage that results in your stomach taking too long to empty; symptoms are nausea, vomiting, and bloating. Nerve damage from diabetes is the most common cause.

Globulins—proteins in your blood that are involved in many functions. Some act as enzymes that trigger chemical reactions in your body. Others act as transporters that carry chemicals from one place to another. Yet others are part of your immune system. They are called *globulins* because they are globe-shaped.

Glucose—a simple sugar that is the main source of energy for your body. Digestion breaks all carbohydrates down into glucose. This glucose is carried in your blood to your body's cells, where it is either used for energy or stored. Impaired glucose metabolism is the cause of diabetes.

Glycemic Index (GI)—a dietary index that is used to rank carbohydrates by how quickly and how much they raise blood sugar after they are consumed. Carbohydrates that raise the blood sugar the fastest have the highest Glycemic Index.

H

HDL cholesterol—high-density lipoprotein cholesterol; the good cholesterol. Helps clean your body's blood vessels of plaque and cholesterol buildup.

Heart attack—death of heart muscle cells due to lack of blood flow to your heart muscle through your coronary arteries. Most often caused by a blockage in one or more coronary arteries from high cholesterol or from a piece of plaque that breaks off a vessel wall and cuts off blood flow to your heart muscle. The medical term is *myocardial infarction* or *MI*.

Heart murmur, innocent—an abnormal heart sound heard through a healthcare provider's stethoscope; indicates turbulent blood flow through your heart's valves that does not impair your heart's ability to pump or function normally. An echocardiogram is needed to tell whether a heart murmur is innocent or represents a problem requiring further evaluation and possibly treatment.

Hemoglobin A1c—a component of red blood cells that carries sugar in the blood, used to measure average blood sugar over the previous 3 months to evaluate blood sugar control in people with diabetes.

Hepatitis—inflammation of your liver; may be caused by infection from a virus (hepatitis A, B, or C), from bacteria or parasites, or from drug or alcohol abuse. May cause no symptoms or a sudden illness characterized by an enlarged liver, jaundice (yellowing of your skin and the whites of your eyes), poor appetite, nausea, and abdominal pain.

Homocysteine—an amino acid (a chemical building block of proteins) that is a by-product of normal protein breakdown. High levels of homocysteine are believed to increase your risk of coronary artery disease; the levels can be lowered by treatment with high doses of folic acid and B vitamins.

Hyperglycemia—high levels of sugar in your blood; most often due to diabetes, but sometimes caused by other conditions.

Hypertension—high blood pressure.

Hypoglycemia—low levels of sugar in your blood; usually occurs in diabetics after taking medication and then not eating enough food or skipping meals; sometimes occurs in non-diabetics whose blood sugar falls to abnormally low levels when they skip meals. Can cause sweats, confusion, and even loss of consciousness; also called *insulin shock*.

I

Insulin—a hormone produced in your pancreas that enables your body to move sugar (glucose) out of your bloodstream and into your cells, where it can be used for energy. Not enough insulin or insulin insensitivity is the cause of diabetes.

Insulin sensitizers—medications used in the treatment of diabetes that increase your body's ability to use insulin.

K

Ketones—chemicals that are produced in your liver when your body breaks down fat for energy. If ketones accumulate in your body, they can lead to coma and even death. High levels of ketones are present in uncontrolled diabetes and can lead to the life-threatening condition of *diabetic ketoacidosis* (DKA).

L

LDL cholesterol—low-density lipoprotein cholesterol; called bad cholesterol because it easily enters your blood vessel walls and causes the buildup of plaque. Is a risk factor for *atherosclerosis*. See "Routine Laboratory Tests."

Left ventricular hypertrophy (LVH)—an abnormal enlargement and thickening of the muscular wall of your left ventricle, which pumps blood out of the heart to the rest of your body. Usually caused by long-standing high blood pressure because your heart has to push against the high pressure and your heart, like any muscle, enlarges from the effort. LVH weakens your heart and increases your risk of heart attack and congestive heart failure.

Leptin—a hormone produced by fat cells that signals your brain to decrease appetite and increase the metabolism of stored fat.

Lipoprotein—a carrier protein in your blood for fat and cholesterol; *LDL* (low-density lipoprotein), *HDL* (high-density lipoprotein), and *VLDL* (very low density lipoprotein) are the three most common types.

Liver cirrhosis—disease of your liver in which functioning liver tissue is replaced by scar tissue; it is caused by damage to your liver, most often from alcohol abuse, hepatitis infections, and some drugs. It is not curable, but its progression can be slowed or halted with proper treatment.

Loading dose—a larger-than-normal dose of a medication given to bring your blood level of a drug up to the therapeutic level; examples of drugs that require loading doses are digoxin for the heart, phenytoin (brand name: Dilantin) for seizure disorders, and theophylline for respiratory disease. Certain psychiatric drugs also require loading doses. These types of drugs that require a loading dose are monitored with periodic blood tests to check that the levels in your blood are not too high or too low.

Low blood sugar—also called *hypoglycemia*. Usually occurs in diabetics after taking medication or *insulin* and then not eating enough food or skipping meals; sometimes occurs in non-diabetics whose blood sugar falls to abnormally low levels when they skip meals. Can cause sweats, confusion, and even loss of conscious. Also called *insulin shock*.

LPN—*see Nurse, Licensed Practical.*

LVH—*see left ventricular hypertrophy.*

M

Masked depression—believing physical symptoms are medical problems when, in fact, they are being caused by unrecognized and untreated depression.

Medical Assistant (MA)—healthcare workers found most often in medical offices. MAs perform a wide range of duties under the supervision of a healthcare provider or office manager; they take medical histories and record vital signs, explain treatment procedures, prepare patients for examination, collect and prepare laboratory specimens and perform laboratory tests in the office. MAs also handle many administrative duties answering telephones, greeting patients, and updating and filing patients' medical records. Formal training is not required but is preferred; vocational schools and junior colleges offer programs to those with high school diplomas or the equivalent that offer a certificate or diploma in one year or an associate degree after two years of training. Certification is available but not required.

Mediterranean diet—a nutritional model based on the traditional dietary patterns of countries in the Mediterranean region (Italy, Greece, and Spain). This type of diet has heart-healthy olive oil as its primary fat; is rich in grains (pasta and breads), which are served along with tomatoes, onions, artichokes, eggplants, peas, lentils, chickpeas and fruits; and gets its protein from grilled or steamed chicken and seafood (as opposed to red meat). A glass or two of red wine a day is part of the diet for those without alcohol problems.

Metabolic syndrome—a set of conditions including high triglycerides, low HDL, abdominal obesity, high blood pressure, and insulin insensitivity. This combination creates a very high risk for diabetes, heart disease, vascular disease, sudden heart attack, and stroke; also called *Syndrome X*.

Metabolize—to break down substances to release energy.

Metastasis—the spread of cancer from its original site to other places in the body.

Myalgia—muscle pain.

Myocardial infarction (MI)—*see heart attack.*

Myositis—inflammation of muscle, caused by muscle damage. May be normal, as after unaccustomed exercise, or abnormal, as in medication side effects or diseases *(see rhabdomyolysis)*.

N

Neurotransmitters—chemicals in your brain that transmit messages from one nerve cell to another.

NP—*see Nurse Practitioner.*

Nurse Assistant, Certified (CNA): healthcare workers, unlicensed but certified, who are known by many names including CNA, Nurse Aides, Orderlies, Patient Care Technicians, and Home Health Aides. An important part of the healthcare team, they provide direct, hands-on care to patients in a wide variety of settings. Education depends on the state, and requirements for certification vary anywhere from two weeks of training followed by a test to several months of clinical and classroom training. CNAs work under the supervision of an RN or LPN.

Nurse, Licensed Practical (LPN)—a licensed health professional who works under the supervision of an RN, NP, MD, or DO; education required is a high school diploma and completion of a formal training program at a vocational school or community college that includes supervised clinical instruction. LPNs must also successfully complete a licensing examination. LPNs can perform many basic nursing functions including administering medications. Their scope of practice varies from state to state.

Nurse Practitioner (NP)—a licensed registered nurse with advanced academic and clinical training at the master's or doctoral level. NPs provide both medical and nursing care under their own license. NPs are licensed to give orders, prescribe medications, and direct medical care of patients. Depending on state law, NPs practice either independently or in collaboration with physicians. NP areas of specialization and certification include Family, Adult, Pediatric, Gerontologic, Women's Health, Psychiatric, School and Occupational Health, Emergency, Neonatal, and Acute Care. NP education is shorter than physician education, and continuing education for certified NPs is 150 hours every five years and recertification is every five years. [See page 251 for more about NP practice.]

Nurse, Registered (RN)—a licensed health professional who is a graduate nurse who has passed an examination for registration. An RN diagnoses human responses to actual and potential health problems. Education required is an Associate's or a Bachelor's degree but may be a Master's or Doctorate degree. RNs provide nursing care, administer medications, provide health counseling and teaching, and supervise less skilled personnel. The RN must have an order to administer medications or give treatments. RNs are not licensed to give orders, prescribe medications, or direct the medical care of patients.

P

PA—*see Physician Assistant.*

Pancreatitis—inflammation of your pancreas, an organ in your abdomen that makes *insulin* and digestive enzymes. Has many causes, but the most common are alcohol abuse and gallstones. Causes severe abdominal pain, nausea, and vomiting.

Peripheral neuropathy—nerve damage that affects the nerves of your arms, legs, hands, and feet and that causes burning, tingling, numbness, weakness, and / or pain. Most common cause is uncontrolled diabetes, but can also be caused by other diseases including HIV, by medications, and by nutritional deficiencies.

Peripheral vascular disease (PVD)—a form of *atherosclerosis* that results in blockages and impaired circulation to your extremities, most often in your legs. Can cause pain with walking (often relieved with rest) because your blood vessels are not able to supply enough blood and oxygen to the muscles of your legs.

Physician (MD or DO)—a licensed health professional (either a Medical Doctor or Doctor of Osteopathy) who provides medical or surgical care in an area of specialization according to the laws of the state in which they practice. Physicians have four years of post-graduate medical education plus two or more years of internship. Licensure is maintained through continuing education of 50 hours per year.

Most MDs and DOs are certified in their area of medical or surgical specialty. MDs and DOs have equivalent education and training—the difference is in their philosophies—DOs tend to be more holistic and preventive in their approach and have additional training in physical manipulation, while MDs tend to be more disease- and medication-focused. DOs are more often found in primary care while most, but not all, specialists are MDs.

Physician Assistant (PA)—a licensed health professional who provides medical care under the supervision of a physician. Training is through accredited formal education programs at either the bachelor's or the master's level and completion of a national certifying examination. Practice is under the license of the supervising physician. PAs have no education or training in nursing. PA education is shorter than physician education and PAs are not required to complete an internship or residency. Licensure is maintained through continuing education of 100 hours every two years and recertification exams every six years.

Plaque—deposits of fat and cholesterol inside the linings of your blood vessels; a characteristic of *atherosclerosis*.

Polycystic ovary syndrome—a hereditary disease characterized by multiple cysts on your ovaries, obesity, excessive hairiness, infertility, irregular menstruation, and cholesterol abnormalities.

Polypharmacy—an excessive number of medications that, instead of working together to improve your health and lower your risks, work at cross-purposes and result in side effects and drug-to-drug interactions.

Purines—chemicals in certain foods that your body metabolizes into uric acid; eating these foods can give you attacks of gout. Foods high in purines include alcohol (especially beer), sweetbreads, anchovies, sardines, liver, herring, mackerel, scallops, game meat, and gravy.

R

Renal arteries—arteries that supply oxygen-rich blood to your kidneys; the two renal arteries pump 1 liter of blood per minute to your two kidneys. Blockage of your renal arteries by *atherosclerosis* can cause high blood pressure, thus increasing your risk of stroke.

Rhabdomyolysis—a life-threatening condition in which destruction of your skeletal muscle results in release of a chemical called myoglobin into your bloodstream; that release in turn can lead to kidney damage and death. Symptoms include severe muscle pain and dark-colored urine; caused by physical damage to your muscle from major trauma, high fever, electrical shock, uncontrolled convulsions, and certain medications.

RN—*see Nurse, Registered.*

S

SBP—*see systolic blood pressure.*

Stents—straw-shaped devices that are placed on a balloon catheter and used to enlarge and keep open narrowed blood vessels.

Stroke—a rupture or blockage of a blood vessel in your brain that prevents blood from reaching part of your brain. The result is injury or death of brain tissue, also called a *brain attack* or *CVA* (cerebrovascular accident).

Synapses—spaces between one nerve cell and another in your brain; at synapses, neurotransmitters are released from one cell and cause the cell on the other side of the synapse to react.

Systolic blood pressure (SBP)—the top number in a blood pressure reading; it represents the highest pressure in your blood vessels that occurs when your heart beats.

T

Target—a reference point to reach in order to reduce your health risk; a goal intended to be attained.

Target organ—an organ in your body that sustains damage from uncontrolled health risk factors; for example, your kidneys may be damaged from high blood pressure.

Transient ischemic attack (TIA)—a cerebrovascular accident, like a stroke, but one that lasts only minutes to hours and resolves without causing permanent damage or disability; also called a *mini-stroke.*

Triglycerides—fats that circulate in your bloodstream that are increased by eating fatty foods and decreased by eating a low-fat diet; high triglycerides can be genetic and are a characteristic of *metabolic syndrome.*

V

Varicella—the virus that causes chickenpox and shingles.

Vascular disease—disease of your blood vessels.

Nurse Practitioner: FAQs

What is a Nurse Practitioner?

A nurse practitioner (NP) is a registered nurse with advanced education and clinical training who delivers the same primary healthcare that doctors do. NPs diagnose, treat, prescribe, and manage acute and chronic illness, just like doctors. But NPs practice from a different perspective than doctors do. That is because our expertise is grounded in our nursing background. NP practice focuses on individualized care with an emphasis on prevention, wellness, and patient education. NPs are noted for spending more time with patients. We do this in order to establish trusting relationships and learn about our patients' preferences and lives. NPs excel at health teaching, managing acute and chronic disease, and coordinating complicated and complex treatment plans among multiple providers. NP care is focused comprehensively on the whole person rather than on a single particular problem.

Is an NP a doctor's assistant?

No, that is a Physician Assistant (PA). Sometimes the two roles are confused, but we are not the same. A Physician Assistant (PA) is by definition trained to be an assistant to a physician. PAs practice under the license of their supervising physician and have no nursing background or training. NPs practice under their own license and are nurse experts who also practice medicine. NPs practice either independently or in collaboration with a physician, depending on the laws of the state in which they work and the experience of the individual NP. In 23 states, NPs may practice independently without physician involvement. In 28 states, NPs practice under a collaborative agreement with a physician who is available to take referrals or offer consultations at the NP's request. (See the Glossary for more on NP, PA, and MD / DOs scopes of practice and training.)

What education and licensing do NP's have?

NPs are titled three ways—by education, by specialty, and by certification.

Education / Licensure: All NPs are now educated with at least a post-graduate master's degree. Clinical doctorate degrees are now being offered and NPs who have completed these programs are titled DNP (Doctor of Nursing Practice). NP titles vary state to state (confusing, but that's how they've done it) and include ARNP (Advanced Registered Nurse Practitioner), APN (Advanced Practice Nurse), APRN (Advanced Practice Registered Nurse), CRNP (Certified Registered Nurse Practitioner), RNP (Registered Nurse Practitioner), and CNP (Certified Nurse Practitioner).

Specialties: NPs are educated by specialty as are physicians. NP areas of specialty are FNP (Family Nurse Practitioner), ANP (Adult Nurse Practitioner), PNP (Pediatric Nurse Practitioner), GNP (Geriatric Nurse Practitioner), WHNP / NPWH (Women's Health Nurse Practitioner), Psych NP (Psychiatric Nurse Practitioner), ACNP (Acute Care Nurse Practitioner), and NNNP (Neonatal Nurse Practitioner). Other areas of specialty include School, Community, Occupational, and Holistic Health Nurse Practitioners. In addition to NPs, other Advanced Practice Nurse specialties include Clinical Nurse Specialists, Nurse Anesthetists, and Nurse Midwives.

Certification: The American Nurses Credentialing Center, which is an arm of the American Nurses Association, and the American Academy of Nurse Practitioners both certify NPs. This is done by examination after graduation from an accredited educational institution and by continuing education for practicing NPs who are already certified.

How does NP care compare with physician care?

There have been over 100 studies of NP practice by both nursing and medicine, and not a single one has shown any negative impact on patients or patients' healthcare when NP care has been compared with physician care. NP care has been shown to be equivalent to and, in some cases, even superior to physician care. NPs receive consistently high marks for patient satisfaction in every study done to date.

If you want to look at some of these studies, they can be found on the

Internet at: http://www.nursingadvocacy.org/faq/apn_md_relative_merits.html.

Nurse Practitioner practice will continue to grow and evolve just as healthcare continues to evolve in order to meet the needs of those it serves.

If this book has revealed nothing else, it has shown that there are many roads up the mountain and many different guides who can help you reach the summit. If you will surround yourself with people you trust, you will reach your destination and have a safer and more pleasant journey. So how do you know whom to choose? Trust yourself and your instincts first. If you do that, you will know when you are being cared for by a professional you can trust.

About the Author

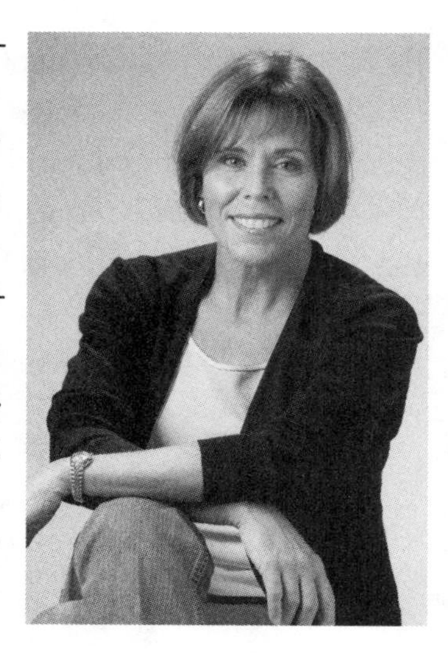

CARLA MILLS, ARNP, completed her undergraduate studies at the Hunter-Bellevue School of Nursing in New York City. She began her nursing career at Bellevue Hospital in the Emergency Department where she became a certified emergency nurse (CEN). Her experience at Bellevue included the general ER, the ER intensive care unit (ICU), and trauma unit. She rounded out her critical care experience at Beekman Downtown Hospital where she worked in the coronary care unit, recovery room, and the medical ICU before leaving New York for Ft. Myers, Florida, in 1989.

Carla expanded her scope of practice from critical care into home healthcare and rehabilitation nursing before returning to graduate school to become a Nurse Practitioner. She completed her Master of Science degree (MSN) at the University of South Florida in Tampa in 1995 and was board-certified as a Family Nurse Practitioner shortly thereafter. Since moving to Naples, Carla has worked in private practice, at Naples Community Hospital in the Emergency Department, and at Naples Urgent Care, a walk-in clinic. She spent three years managing the medical care of patients seeking inpatient treatment for substance abuse and eating disorder problems at the Willough at Naples Psychiatric Hospital prior to joining the practice of Dr. Diane Brzezinski where she currently practices.

Carla has written this book on health risks specifically for patients with no prior medical knowledge. She has also designed a computer database that enables both individuals and health professionals to identify individual health risks as well as track and measure their reduction. Carla believes that the very best healthcare occurs before there is illness and that the very best care of all is self-care.

❖ ❖ ❖

Acknowledgements

This book would not exist but for the generosity of a small army of highly skilled professionals who have given generously of their time and expertise to help make it happen. I am so fortunate to have had their wisdom and support in bringing this book to completion.

I will be forever indebted to my writing partner, yoga teacher, and good friend, Jamie Shane. At my invitation, she bravely took an unwieldy manuscript and injected it with as much of her formidable literary charm as she could muster. She did a fantastic job and has helped its readability enormously. Thanks, Jamie.

I want to acknowledge and thank the following extraordinary Nurse Practitioners for their input, advice, and peer reviews over the 10 years the project has been in development: my professional role model, Cyndie Grimes, as well as Lillian Tibbles, Niki Saltzer, Bonnie Bodin, Noelle Kauramaki, W. Lane Edwards, Jr., and my friend, Germaine Eurich, who provided essential research and moral support just when it was needed most.

I have learned so much from and am so grateful to the following Registered Nurses. They are the best of the best and taught me by their example how the art of nursing is practiced: Julie Hall, Diane Smith, Melanie Simmons, Meri Shaffer, and Erika Hinson.

Very special thanks are owed to the nurses in the Emergency Department at Bellevue Hospital in New York City. That is where I was trained and where my nursing career began. I still cherish the guidance and wisdom I received from my mentors, Joyce Buffolino and Elizabeth Reynolds Chiappe—they are without doubt the two greatest nurses in the universe. Other nurses I was privileged to work alongside and learn from are Joann Belmont, Rose Marie Caciolla, Tom Carlo, Joanne Croke, Eileen Davis, Sue Draper, Meredith Altman Flomenbaum, Holly Hartung, Eileen Houlihan, Ed Kearns, Rhonda Krinsky, Danielle and Walter La Strange, Annette Hunter Lisecki, Marion Machado, Esther Magid, Sue Callahan Montella, Helen Murphy, Sherri Rappaport Nodelman, Kathy O'Donnell, Helen Ornstein, Charlene Petrec, Pat Sorenson, Jean McGowan Starace, Elizabeth Swanson, Ann Marie Ward, and Lisa Wing.

My grateful thanks to the following physicians: To the late Dr. Thomas Brittingham, Sr., thanks for believing I could grow into what I have become … and for continuing even now to sit on my shoulder whispering sage advice in my ear whenever my knowledge or courage falters. To Dr. Robert Boyd Tober, you're the best doctor I've worked with of your generation and a true hero; you should be Surgeon General of this country. Thank you for sharing your visionary intelligence and for your steady support and enthusiasm for this project from its very beginning—including writing the book's Foreword. To Dr. Robert Statfeld, thank you for being there when the going was toughest. Your loyalty, good humor, and unwavering commitment to doing the right thing, regardless of the outcome, mattered then and still does. And, finally, to Dr. Diane Brzezinski, the physician with whom I practice, thank you for making a home for me and for allowing me to share in the care of your patients. Your keen mind, sharp diagnostic skills, and loving heart have created a rare safe haven of medical care in a world where it is often hard to find. And aren't we lucky to have the nicest patients it has been my pleasure to care for in 20 plus years of practice?

This book would not have been published were it not for helpful editorial advice offered at various stages along the way. Thanks to Elizabeth Zack at Bookcrafters for tackling the first professional edit of the material. Heartfelt thanks to my childhood friend, Draper Shreeve, for offering early advice and direction when the book was first being conceived.

But without Jennifer McCord and her associates, the book would have certainly withered and died on the vine. Editorial advice and development offered by Roberta Trahan and Gloria D. Campbell were essential to rounding off the book's rough edges. Design work by Jeanie James gave the manuscript wings to fly and offers a warm invitation to readers to take a chance on the journey. Medical proofing by Susan London corrected errors and verified accuracy. In order for readers with health concerns to find the information they need, Kathryn Shield of Colleen Dunham Indexing carefully read and distilled the material and wrote an exhaustive and easy-to-use index.

And the most special thanks of all go to Jennifer McCord herself. Jennifer, you cannot know how much you are appreciated. Through this long, long process of turning a manuscript into a book, whenever I needed anything you were there. Thank you for never telling me what I wanted to hear. Thank you for sticking with the project. Thank you for never dropping a single email. Thank you for listening and being a friend.

Acknowledgements cannot be complete without thanking family and close friends for their faithful and loving support through the years this book has been in development and all the years that preceded it.

First in line for thanks is my sister, Vicki Mills, and her company Concord Web Solutions. Vicki has been my most trusted and respected advisor from earliest conception of this book. Not only is Vicki one of the smartest people I know, she is also a bright and discerning literary, design, and marketing critic. Her editorial and critical input was always offered with the gentleness of a loving sister and best friend. Without her this book could never have happened—thanks, Vick!

Thanks, too, are owed to my brother, David Mills, Jr., for sharing his entrepreneurial spirit, to my late parents, Marge Miller Mills and David E. Mills, Sr., for, well, everything, and to my step-mother, Betty Mills, for her loyalty, kindness, love, and generosity in all things.

Finally, I would not be here to write about health and the pursuit of happiness were it not for my two best friends and their families. Without them I could never have grown up healthy, and because of them I was lucky enough to grow up happy. To Connie Heard Meyer, my best friend since third grade, husband Edgar, son George, Connie's parents Jean and Alexander Heard, brothers Stephen, Christopher, and Frank and their families—thanks for always being there for me and for my family. To Margaret Brittingham Brant, husband Kevin, sons Matthew and Robert, parents Dotsy and Tom Brittingham, brothers and sisters Johnny, Susie, Harold, Tommy, and Sally and their families—thanks for letting me into your family whom I love as dearly as I love my own.

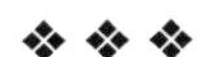

Index

D

E

F

G

J

K

L

M

N

O

Photo credits:

Author photos:	Robert Nelson Photography
Chapter photos:	
How Is Your Health?	www.bigstockphoto.com ©Lee Seoul
User Guide	www.istockphoto.com ©Ralph Hoppe
Knowing Is Half the Battle	www.istockphoto.com
Are You at Risk?	www.bigstockphoto.com ©Jane Brennecker
What Are Your Risks?	www.istockphoto.com ©Steve Harmon
Medications and Your Health	www.fotolia.com ©Marcel Liebenberg
Your First Choice: Exercise	www.fotolia.com ©Mark Ross
Your Second Choice: Weight and Nutrition	www.bigstockphoto.com ©Simone van den Berg
Your Third Choice: Mental Resilience	www.istockphoto.com ©Garrett Bautista
Change: How to Stick to Your Choices	www.istockphoto.com ©Y. Yang
Good Health in a Nutshell	www.fotolia.com ©T. Wojnarowicz
A Final Pep Talk.	www.istockphoto.com ©John Carleton
Postscript	www.bigstockphoto.com ©Andres Rodriguez